ADVANCE PRAISE FOR
The Raw Milk Revolution

"David Gumpert employs his expertise as a professional business writer to dig deep and wide into the exploding raw milk controversy. His compelling analysis of the science, economics, politics and history of 'nature's most perfect food' opens the door to a greater understanding of the major challenges facing our food and agriculture systems today. Anyone concerned with the health of our people, our environment, and our democracy should heed his words."

—DEAN FLOREZ, Majority Leader,
California State Senate

"If you want to understand the vocal opposition to food safety laws, you should read Gumpert's book. That's not the only reason to read it, though. Even if you have little interest in raw milk, I think this book is a key piece in the puzzle to understanding the backwards priorities in America's food-safety system."

—JILL RICHARDSON, founder of
La Vida Locavore.org and author
of *Recipe for America*

"David Gumpert has chronicled the Raw Milk War with insight and humor. He provides an important record of systematic government bias against Nature's perfect food. Must reading for raw milk fans and government officials alike."

—SALLY FALLON MORELL, President,
The Weston A. Price Foundation

"David Gumpert has become the official chronicler of the 'raw milk movement' in the United States. *The Raw Milk Revolution* is a highly readable exposé that successfully captures how the controversy over raw milk is at the center of a larger battle between the industrial food system and the local food movement. Gumpert explains how raw milk, more than any other food, threatens proponents of the 'germ theory,' centralized food production, and the 'nanny state.' *The Raw Milk Revolution* is an extremely important book because it sounds a clear warning that upholding the right to produce and consume raw milk is critical in preserving our food freedoms in general."

—PETER KENNEDY, President,
Farm-to-Consumer Legal Defense Fund

THE RAW MILK
REVOLUTION

THE RAW MILK REVOLUTION

*Behind America's Emerging
Battle Over Food Rights*

David E. Gumpert

Foreword by
JOEL SALATIN

CHELSEA GREEN PUBLISHING
WHITE RIVER JUNCTION, VERMONT

Project Manager: Emily Foote
Developmental Editor: Benjamin Watson
Copy Editor: Laura Jorstad
Proofreader: Emily Foote
Indexer: Shana Milkie
Designer: Peter Holm, Sterling Hill Productions

Printed in the United States of America
First printing November 2009
10 9 8 7 6 5 4 3 2 1   09 10 11 12 13 14

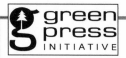

Chelsea Green Publishing is committed to preserving ancient forests and natural resources. We elected to print this title on 30-percent postconsumer recycled paper, processed chlorine-free. As a result, for this printing, we have saved:

12 Trees (40' tall and 6-8" diameter)
5,305 Gallons of Wastewater
4 Million BTUs Total Energy
322 Pounds of Solid Waste
1,101 Pounds of Greenhouse Gases

Chelsea Green Publishing made this paper choice because we and our printer, Thomson-Shore, Inc., are members of the Green Press Initiative, a nonprofit program dedicated to supporting authors, publishers, and suppliers in their efforts to reduce their use of fiber obtained from endangered forests. For more information, visit: www.greenpressinitiative.org.

Environmental impact estimates were made using the Environmental Defense Paper Calculator. For more information visit: www.papercalculator.org.

Our Commitment to Green Publishing

Chelsea Green sees publishing as a tool for cultural change and ecological stewardship. We strive to align our book manufacturing practices with our editorial mission and to reduce the impact of our business enterprise on the environment. We print our books and catalogs on chlorine-free recycled paper, using vegetable-based inks whenever possible. This book may cost slightly more because we use recycled paper, and we hope you'll agree that it's worth it. Chelsea Green is a member of the Green Press Initiative (www.greenpressinitiative.org), a nonprofit coalition of publishers, manufacturers, and authors working to protect the world's endangered forests and conserve natural resources.

The Raw Milk Revolution was printed on Natures Natural, a 30-percent postconsumer recycled paper supplied by Thomson-Shore.

Library of Congress Cataloging-in-Publication Data
Gumpert, David E.
   The raw milk revolution : behind America's emerging battle over food rights / David E. Gumpert ; foreword by Joel Salatin.
     p. ; cm.
   Includes bibliographical references and index.
   ISBN 978-1-60358-219-3
   1. Milk--Microbiology--United States. 2. Bacterial diseases--Prevention. 3. Medical policy--United States. 4. Food law and legislation--United States. 5. Milk--Sterlization--Law and legislation--United States. I. Title.
   [DNLM: 1. Milk--United States. 2. Bacterial Infections--prevention & control--United States. 3. Health Policy--United States. 4. Legislation, Food--United States. 5. Milk--microbiology--United States. 6. Sterilization--legislation & jurisprudence--United States. WA 719 G974r 2009]

QR121.G86 2009
363.19'29--dc22

                                        2009031406

Chelsea Green Publishing Company
Post Office Box 428
White River Junction, VT 05001
(802) 295-6300
www.chelseagreen.com

DEDICATION

This book is dedicated to the dairy farmers across the U.S. who brave government interference and harassment to produce safe raw milk for the many consumers committed to exercising their right to consume the foods of their choice.

CONTENTS

I drink raw milk, sold illegally on the underground black market. I grew up on raw milk from our own Guernsey cows that our family hand-milked twice a day. We made yogurt, ice cream, butter, and cottage cheese. All through high school in the early 1970s, I sold our homemade yogurt, butter, buttermilk, and cottage cheese at the Curb Market on Saturday mornings. This was a precursor to today's farmer's markets.

In those days, the Virginia Department of Agriculture had a memorandum of agreement with the Curb Market that as long as vendors belonged to an Agricultural Extension organization such as Extension Homemaker's Clubs or 4-H, producers could bring value-added products to market without inspection and visits from the food police. The government agents assumed that anyone participating in the extension programs would be getting the latest, greatest food science and therefore conform to the most modern procedural protocols, which created its own protection.

As the Virginia Slims commercial says, "We've come a long way, baby." These conciliatory overtures to maintain healthy and vibrant local food economies exist no more. Today I can't sell any of those things at a farmer's market, and even if I take eggs some bureaucrat will come along with a pocket thermometer and, without warrant or warning, reach over and poke it through my display eggs to see if they are at the proper temperature. If they aren't, no amount of pleading that those are for display only can dissuade the petulant public servant from demanding that I dump those display eggs in a trash can on the spot. I don't sell at farmer's markets anymore.

In 1975, when I graduated from high school and began plotting my farming career, I figured out that I could hand-milk ten cows, sell the milk to neighbors at regular retail prices, and be a full-time farmer. This was before most people had ever heard the word *organic*. But selling milk was illegal. In those days, we didn't know about herd shares or Community Supported Agriculture or even limited liability corporations.

As a result, I went to work for a local newspaper and became the proverbial part-time farmer—working in town to support the farming passion. I don't think I've ever gotten over the fact that the government arbitrarily determined to make it very difficult for me to become a farmer. That seems un-American, doesn't it?

Isn't it curious that at this juncture in our culture's evolution, we collectively believe Twinkies, Lucky Charms, and Coca-Cola are safe foods, but compost-grown tomatoes and raw milk are not. With legislation moving through Congress demanding that all agricultural practices be "science-based," I believe our food system is at Wounded Knee. I do not believe that is an overstatement.

Make no mistake, as the local, heritage, humane, ecological, sustainable—call it what you will (anything but organic since the government now owns that word)—food system takes flight, the industrial food system is fighting back. With a vengeance. By demonizing, criminalizing, and marginalizing the integrity food movement, the entrenched powers that be hope to derail this revolution.

This industrial food experiment, historically speaking, is completely abnormal. It's not normal to eat things you can't spell or pronounce. It's not normal to eat things you can't make in your kitchen. Indeed, if everything in today's science-based supermarket that was unavailable before 1900 were removed, hardly anything would be left. And as more people realize that this grand experiment in ingesting material totally foreign to our three-trillion-member internal community of intestinal microflora and -fauna is really biologically aberrant behavior, they are opting out of industrial fare. Indeed, to call it a food revolution is accurate.

But revolutions are always met with prejudice and entrenched paradigms from the about-to-be-unseated lords of the status quo. The realignment of power, trust, money, and commerce that the local heritage-based food movement represents inherently gives birth to a backlash. By the time of Wounded Knee, Native Americans no longer jeopardized the American reality.

But to many Americans, these Natives had to be crushed, extinguished, put on reservations. Would America have been stronger if European leaders had listened to wisdom about herbal remedies and consensus building? The answer is yes. But to Americans, the red man was just a barbarian because he didn't govern by parliamentary procedure or ride in horse-drawn stagecoaches along cobblestone streets. In fact, he was considered a threat to America. Just like giving slaves their freedom in 1850. Just like imbibing alcohol in 1925. Just like homeschooling in 1980.

The ultimate test of a tyrannical society or a free society is how it responds to its lunatic fringe. A strong, self-confident, free society tolerates and enjoys the fringe people who come up with zany notions. Indeed, most people later labeled geniuses were dubbed whacko by their contemporary mainstream society. So what does a culture do with weirdos who actually believe they have a right to choose what to feed their internal three-trillion-member community?

The only reason the right to food choice was not guaranteed in the Bill of Rights is because the Founders of America could not have envisioned a day when selling a glass of raw milk or homemade pickles to a neighbor would be outlawed. At the time, such a thought was as strange as levitation.

Indeed, what good is the freedom to own guns, worship, or assemble if we don't have the freedom to eat the proper fuel to energize us to shoot, pray, and preach? Is not freedom to choose our food at least as fundamental a right as the freedom to worship?

How would we feel if we had to get a license from bureaucrats to start a church? After all, beliefs can be pretty damaging things. And charlatans certainly do exist. Better protect people from those charlatans—bad preachers and raw milk advocates.

But what does a society do when the charlatans are in charge? In charge of the regulating government agencies. In charge of the research institutions. In charge of the food system.

That is a real conundrum, because if health depends on opting out of what the charlatans think is safe, we are forced into civil disobedience. When the public no longer trusts its public servants, people begin taking charge of their own health and welfare. And that is exactly what is driving the local heritage food movement.

Lots of folks realize they don't want industrialists fooling around with something as basic as food. People like me don't trust Monsanto. We don't trust the Food and Drug Administration. We don't trust the Department of Agriculture. We don't trust Tyson. And we don't think it's safe to be dependent on food that sits for a month in the belly of a Chinese merchant marine vessel.

This clash of choice versus prohibition brings us to today's Wounded Knee of food. The local heritage-based food movement represents everything that is good and noble about farming and food culture. It is about decentralized farms. Pastoral livestock systems. Symbiotic multi-speciation. Companion planting. Earthworms. It is about community-appropriate techniques and scale. Aesthetically and aromatically sensual romantic farming. Re-embedding the butcher, baker, and candlestick maker in the village. And ultimately about health-giving food grown more productively on less land than industrial models.

Certainly some of this clash represents the difference between nurturing and dominating. The local heritage food movement—the raw milk movement—is all about respecting and honoring indigenous wisdom. The industrial mind-set worships techno-glitzy gadgetry and views heritage food advocates as simpletons and Luddites. Or dangerous criminals.

In this wonderful exposé, David Gumpert employs the best journalistic investigative techniques to examine this clash from the raw milk battlefront. Be assured that the same mentality exists toward homemade pickles, home-cured meats, and cottage industry in general. The entrepreneurial spirit is alive and well in the food system, but it is harassed out of existence by capricious, malicious, and prejudiced government agents who really do believe they are doing society a favor by denying food choice to Americans.

The same curative properties espoused by raw milk advocates exist in a host of other food products, from homemade pound cake and potpies to pepperoni and pastured chicken. Real food is what developed our internal intestinal community. And it sure didn't develop on food from Concentrated Animal Feeding Operations and genetically modified potatoes that are partly human and partly tomato. Long after human cleverness has run its course, compost piles will still grow the best tomatoes and grazing cows will still yield one of nature's perfect foods: raw milk.

One of our former apprentices has just started a ten-cow herd-share arrangement with our customers. Here is a young, entrepreneurial, go-get-'em farmer embarking on his dream, serving people who are enjoying their dream of acquiring unadulterated milk. Can any arrangement, any relationship—between farmer and cow, cow and pasture, customer and producer—be more honorable, respectable, open, and trusting? Everything about this is righteous, including respecting the individual enough to let her decide what to eat and what to feed her children.

Let the revolution continue.

JOEL SALATIN
Polyface Farm, Swoope, Virginia
June 2009

Why the Sudden Concern About Food Rights?

We Americans have a tendency to take our food for granted. When you walk into a large grocery store, it seems as if there is no food product, no matter how exotic or out of season, that isn't readily available.

Yet as recently as the mid-1980s, if you were wary of all the fruits and vegetables grown with pesticides and factory-produced fertilizers, and wanted organic produce instead, there weren't many options. At the time, Whole Foods Market was just a local phenomenon in Austin, Texas, and there were only a few similar offbeat stores in big cities around the country.

However, as more consumers became concerned about the dangers of our conventional produce and began demanding organic food instead, the market adjusted. Whole Foods morphed into a national chain, farmer's markets sprang up everywhere, and eventually even conventional chains like Wal-Mart began carrying organic produce. In short, the market accommodated to changes in demand.

Today growing numbers of consumers are coming to realize that they would like to serve their families raw (unpasteurized) milk. Like the consumers of twenty-five years ago who worried about the integrity of conventional produce, today's consumers worry about the integrity of pasteurized milk and whether it has significant nutritive value. They see in the unpasteurized version access to essential "good" bacteria and enzymes that can help build their immune systems and improve their overall health.

For about two-thirds of the nation's consumers, though, raw milk either is unavailable or requires a drive to a farm that could be an hour or more away from home.

But unlike the rapid growth in the organic food sector, as demand for raw dairy grows, the market will not be able to easily accommodate the change in demand. The reason is that, in the places where raw milk is unavailable or available only on farms, the market choices have been set as a matter of law or regulation. Those laws and regulations have, over the last fifty years, become more rather than less restrictive. And if the US Food and Drug Administration, the federal agency that regulates dairy foods, has its way, unpasteurized milk will be completely outlawed sooner rather than later.

Well, you might say, we're just talking about one narrowly appealing offbeat product. The supermarkets are still well stocked with all kinds of other similar foods. We can take probiotic supplements to obtain at least some of the good bacteria provided by raw milk.

But the fact of the matter is that we aren't talking about just one product. If you want unpasteurized fruit and vegetable juices, which are also thought to contain beneficial enzymes and bacteria, you won't find them in any grocery chains, including Whole Foods. Beginning in the late 1990s, the FDA went after those juice products, and as a result they all must now be pasteurized. You may still find some unpasteurized juices at the occasional farmer's market or farm stand, but in some states, such as New York, even apple cider sold direct by the farmer to the consumer must be pasteurized. And the only unpasteurized vegetable juices are those available from occasional specialty stores that mix them up for you.

If you are a real food aficionado and want to buy your almonds unpasteurized, well, those just bit the dust as well. The California Almond Board, with approval of the US Department of Agriculture, mandated that all California almonds (pretty much the entire American supply) be pasteurized beginning in 2007.

Now let's look ahead ten or twenty years. Let's say you walk into a supermarket and want to buy some fresh spinach, or chicken or beef, but you want to be sure it hasn't been irradiated—fed a low dose of radiation to kill off possible pathogens. You are concerned because you think the radiation may kill off beneficial nutrients in addition. Too bad—all the non-irradiated stuff has been sold. Or, worse, the non-irradiated foods are no longer allowed to be sold. Food irradiation was first permitted in 2000 and took a while to become accepted, but at this point in the future, it's going full-blast. In other words, the non-irradiated food is contraband, just as raw milk is now considered illegal in many areas of the country.

Now let's look ahead a little farther, perhaps twenty or thirty years from today. You want to buy a leg of lamb, or a pork chop, but you don't want it from a cloned sheep or pig. Too bad—the noncloned varieties of meat are only produced by small farms, and there aren't enough small farms to ensure a regular supply. Or maybe the noncloned variety has just been rendered illegal—the FDA, after allowing production in 2008, decided that so-called natural meat had a higher risk of containing pathogens and was just "too risky" for consumption. Too bad.

The Raw Milk Revolution is ostensibly a book concerning the pitched battle's taking place over one seemingly oddball food. But the reason this fight is so emotionally charged is because it's really a battle over endless numbers of other foods as well. As Joel Salatin points out in the Foreword, it's a battle over a right so fundamental and natural that the authors of the Constitution and the Declaration of Independence didn't think to mention it: the right to obtain the foods we feel are healthiest and safest for us and our families, despite what government regulators, public health professionals, and the medical establishment may want us to believe.

ACKNOWLEDGEMENTS

This book was for all practical purposes launched on my blog, www.thecompletepatient.com, when I began reporting on the state and federal crackdown on raw milk in the fall of 2006. Even though I created regular updates and commentaries on the situation that evolved over the next three years, it was hundreds of readers who graced the blog with amazingly insightful commentary who deserve the bulk of the credit for having inspired *The Raw Milk Revolution*.

As you'll see when you read *The Raw Milk Revolution*, it's readers sharing their experiences and insights who make the book come alive. What's been most amazing to me is not so much the diversity of opinions, but the depth of knowledge these individuals have brought to the discussion. Whether they agree or disagree, these are the smartest, most insightful people I have had the privilege to know.

I want to acknowledge, in particular, some of the blog "regulars" who deserve special attention (listed in no special order). I am certain I have left out some individuals, and so I apologize in advance: Dave Milano, Steve Bemis, Miguel, Lykke, Linda Diane Feldt, Blair McMorran, Bob Hayles, Don Wittlinger, Sylvia Gibson, Milk Farmer, Damaged Justice, Concerned Person, Truly Concerned, Bill Marler, Mary McGonigle-Martin, Paul Hubbard, Gwen Elderberry, Elizabeth McInerney, Hugh Betcha, Don Neeper, Mark McAfee, Greg Bravo, Ruth Ann, Regulator, Ken Conrad, Kimberly Hartke, David Kendall, Amanda Rose, Dave Augenstein, and Robert Monahan.

In addition to my bloggers, I want to acknowledge another group of individuals—a small number of ordinary people brave enough to challenge the might of large-government authority, and arrogance. I couldn't have written this book without the cooperation of a number of owners of dairy farmers, who shared their stories with me, despite risk of retribution from the agriculture departments that police them. You'll meet them in my book—they include Gary Oaks of Kentucky; Richard Hebron of Michigan; Carol Schmitmeyer of Ohio; Chuck Phippen, Lori and Darren McGrath, Dawn Sharts, and Barb and Steve Smith--all of New York; and finally, Ron Garthwaite and Collette Cassidy, as well as Mark McAfee of California

I'm also indebted to a few government scientists and regulators who generously agreed to be interviewed, and answer questions on the science and policy issues raised in this book. One has been Michele Jay-Russell, a researcher at the Western Institute for Food Safety and Security at the University of California, Davis. As a public health professional who has had wide experience in uncovering and assessing food-borne illness, she was able to provide perspective on how problems with raw milk compare with those in other foods. Thanks also to Lewis Jones, chief of the Ohio Department of Agriculture's Dairy Division, who was more open in answering my questions, to the point of including painful personal experiences, than just about any other regulator I dealt with.

I want to especially thank as well two organizations that have been front and center in fighting the government's crackdown. First is the Weston A. Price Foundation, and its director, Sally Fallon Morell. The WAPF has countered propaganda from the U.S. Food and Drug Administration and the U.S. Centers for Disease Control with its own interpretations of scientific papers, as well as provided regular news updates about dairy farmers in trouble with government agencies for distributing raw milk. I don't agree with all its interpretations of research or possible illness from raw dairy, but I admire its willingness to stand up to heavy-handed government initiatives designed to intimidate the farm and research communities, and to encourage undue fear in consumers.

The second organization is the Farm-to-Consumer Legal Defense Fund. It was established July 4, 2007, by a number of individuals with connections to the Weston A. Price Foundation. It was established to provide legal advice and legal assistance to farmer members seeking to establish herd-share and other such arrangements that allow them to distribute raw milk and other nutrient-dense foods to the growing number of individuals seeking them.

The FTCLDF has also represented in court actions dairy farmers accused of wrongdoing for distributing raw dairy products. It has challenged as well a number of government initiatives seen as unfair to smaller farms in general—such as the National Animal Identification System (NAIS), which seeks the registration of billions of farm animals, and would place a heavy burden on small farms. Pete Kennedy, Gary Cox, Tim Wightman, and Cathy Raymond have been tireless in pursuing these cases, and despite working seemingly endless hours, have always made themselves available to answer my questions and provide me with important documentation for my reporting and investigations.

Related to these organizations are two individuals active on behalf of raw milk. Steve Bemis, a lawyer, and Ted Beals, a retired pathologist, both based in Michigan, have similarly helped explain complex legal cases and research.

Thanks to Joel Salatin, the Virginia farmer, who generously agreed to write the book's foreword. Joel is a strong and articulate voice on behalf of food rights, and I am honored that he agreed to introduce the issues surrounding the struggle over raw milk. I also want to thank Nick Leiber, the small business editor at BusinessWeek.com, and Joan Connell, the former online editor of *The Nation*, for helping make possible a number of articles I wrote about the legal and regulatory problems facing raw dairy farmers.

I want to acknowledge as well a number of people who worked behind the scenes to make this book happen. There's my agent, Jennifer Unter of The Unter Agency in New York, who was always available with wise counsel. I was fortunate as well to be able to work with the editors at Chelsea Green Publishing Co. in White River Junction, VT—all of whom understand well the important legal and rights issues at the heart of this story. It was a joy to work with Ben Watson, who did the primary editing, for both his knowledge of food issues, as well as his ideas and insights for improving the book's readability. Emily Foote managed the entire process, and Laura Jorstad smoothed the text out with expert copy editing. Because they truly believe in the emerging importance of food rights, they have demonstrated the sort of commitment to quality that I have never before seen in a commercial book publisher. They walk the walk. Another key behind-the-scenes person was Shana Milkie, an indexer in Ann Arbor, MI, who worked with me on the tedious chore of making sure endnotes were accurately and properly presented.

In completing this kind of project, a writer inevitably neglects family and friends—my thanks to my wife, Jean, and my children (Jason and Laura) and their spouses (Kelly and Jeremy) for their understanding as I closeted myself in the final months to complete this book. I also want to thank my good friend, Leonard Finn, a family practice physician, who patiently answered my questions about the science and realities of various pathogens and chronic conditions.

Why Raw Milk So Inflames the Passions

In 2006, several of America's largest states—Michigan, California, New York, Ohio, and Pennsylvania, in coordination with the US government—launched a major enforcement campaign to crack down on small dairies producing and distributing unpasteurized milk. The campaign was ostensibly designed to accomplish three goals:

- Find suspected pathogens in the growing quantities of unpasteurized milk being consumed in the US.
- Use the findings to warn Americans about the dangers of consuming unpasteurized milk.
- Discourage small dairies from switching their production from conventional milk intended for pasteurization to milk intended for sale and human consumption without being pasteurized.

This book is the story of that campaign—its unusual tactics and surprising findings and outcomes, as seen through the eyes of government officials, scientists, milk producers, and consumers. As such, it's neither a pretty nor a pleasant story. In and of itself, it's a disturbing account of arrogant and insulated regulators running roughshod over the rights of both small farmers and health-conscious consumers. It's also the story of a debate that has been raging for more than a hundred years, but has reintensified because of the government's assault on producers of raw milk.

If the story of the government's actions and the resulting debate were just about raw milk, with an estimated 1 to 3 percent of the milk market, it would be a curiosity, but not necessarily all that important. It turns out, however, that the controversy over raw milk relates to a number of larger issues: the vast changes that have occurred in American agriculture, specifically the way in which our food is produced and distributed on an industrial scale; and the growing concerns over explosive rates of chronic disease, highly publicized outbreaks of food-borne illness, and increasing government involvement and regulation of the foods we eat, as well as the forms in which we are allowed to purchase and consume them. As such, the story of the government's campaign against a nearly forgotten basic food reveals a public policy born of fear and misinformation—one that, in the end, promises to affect the lives of many millions of Americans.

When I was a boy growing up in the 1950s and 1960s, my family would take long cross-country auto trips from our home in Chicago. To distract my sister and me from fighting, my parents would encourage the two of us to count cows among the seemingly endless herds grazing the countryside. With just a few exceptions, like the deserts of Utah and Nevada, or the mountains of Colorado, it didn't matter where we were, because there always seemed to be plenty of cows. So many that the game usually grew boring very quickly.

Today you would be hard-pressed to find even a few cows as you travel America's highways. In many places, including traditional dairy-producing states like Vermont, New York, and Pennsylvania, you generally have to get yourself onto true backcountry roads before you have even a chance of viewing the pastoral landscape of cows grazing on real grass, or crowding under large oak trees to escape the summer sun.

This doesn't mean there are all that many fewer cows around—over the thirty-six-year period beginning in 1970, the number of dairy cows in the United States fell just 19 percent.[1] It just means they have, shall we say, been reorganized. California is now the nation's largest dairy state, but the reason you tend not to see many cows grazing there is that they have been moved from expansive pastures into much smaller factory-style feedlot operations, which you can catch a glimpse of here and there as you drive in the Sacramento area and through the state's vast Central Valley.

In effect, what's happened is that small dairies with a few hundred acres of pasture have gradually disappeared, unable to make dairy farming work economically in a highly regulated, commodity-based economy where the wholesale prices paid for milk often don't even cover the cost of feed, not to mention yielding income to the owners. The statistics testify to these changes. Between 1970 and 2006, the number of farms with dairy cows fell an astounding 88 percent, from 648,000 to 75,000, according to the US Department of Agriculture.[2]

The loss of the small dairy farm—a trend that's been under way since the 1950s—has always seemed like a terrible tragedy to me. And I always assumed the government agreed with me, since presidential candidates campaigning in primary contests in Iowa and New Hampshire invariably talk about helping small farms remain economically viable.

But then I began researching the problems associated with raw milk, and found out different. As I learned about ever more outrageous instances of government regulators who had raided small dairies and confiscated their hard-earned milk and cream, and of how the regulators in some cases even subjected the farmers to harsh interrogation and humiliating searches of their homes, I kept waiting for an agriculture official somewhere in one of America's big dairy states—such as California, Michigan, Pennsylvania, Ohio, and New York—to say something to this effect: "You know, we really want to see these small dairies succeed because they are such important components of strong local economies. We don't necessarily approve of people consuming raw milk, but we know how much a part of America's past and tradition are tied up in these kinds of operations. We're going to work with them to see if we can help them do what they want to do within the confines of the law."

I rarely heard anything approaching such statements. The closest came from Pennsylvania agriculture secretary Dennis Wolff, who in 2007 testified at a state senate hearing into raw milk sales:

> Since at least 1935 . . . Pennsylvania has offered dairy farmers the ability to sell raw milk directly to consumers. The demand for—and profitability of—this portion of the retail milk market is rising, as evidenced by the 75 dairy operations who currently hold raw milk permits for sales directly to consumers. The number of raw milk permit applications and permit holders has nearly doubled in the last two years. Combined with our hundreds of pasteurized milk permit holders, the dairy farmers of Pennsylvania as a whole keep striving to meet market demands and remain viable and hopefully profitable.

But he combined such hopeful language with a blunt warning to the growing number of Pennsylvania dairy farmers seeking to organize private buying clubs for consumers that would enable the dairies to also supply higher-margin products such as yogurt, cream, and butter, which aren't allowed under the existing permits that enable farmers to sell fluid raw milk to the general public. Wolff cited the case of one farmer who took this route:

> Because this farmer refused to obtain the required permit, and con-
> tinued to sell a potentially dangerous product, putting consumers

at risk, he left the department no choice but to pursue legal action against him.[3]

More typically, state and federal agriculture officials simply refuse to discuss the issue of raw milk. As I describe later in this book, the US Food and Drug Administration's chief dairy regulator takes pains to avoid even being in the same building with advocates of raw milk. When California's senate in 2008 held widely publicized hearings to consider legislation that would fix some problems in existing laws affecting raw milk, the California Department of Food and Agriculture refused to send a representative to testify, enraging the committee chairman.

Why has there been such intense official intolerance and animosity against a product that the vast majority of people know little or nothing about, and care about even less? The more I researched raw milk and wrote on my blog about the intense conflicts that kept emerging from the government's crackdown, the more I realized that the controversy over raw milk bumps up against three important fault lines in our society.

1. Traditional Versus Factory Farming

When I want raw milk, I drive to a small farm in New Hampshire along the Connecticut River. Kathy, the owner, has three cows, and she'll ask me whether I want milk from Selena or Nora, the two cows then giving milk. She generally advises me to take Selena's milk, since she's a full Guernsey; Nora is three-quarters Guernsey, and her milk doesn't have as much beta-carotene and butterfat content. This is traditional farming, to the extreme.

If I purchased pasteurized milk at the local supermarket, the milk in a single half-gallon would likely have come from one hundred or more cows. It would have been heated to 161 degrees Fahrenheit for fifteen to twenty seconds, its butterfat reduced to make separate cream products, and spun through filters to reduce its fat globules so they wouldn't rise to the top, as they do in conventional milk.

Over the last century, the number of farms overall has declined by more than two-thirds,[4] and most farms today are oriented toward factory-farming techniques—heavy use of fertilizers and pesticides to raise crops and vast feedlots and similar confined spaces for raising dairy cows, pigs, and chickens. We are continually reminded of factory farming's dangers: In mid-2009, a worldwide pandemic of swine flu was thought to have originated in a huge factory pig farm in Mexico. And places like Kathy's New Hampshire farm, where my milk comes from a particular cow, are harder and harder to find.

Ironically, it was huge, disgusting feedlots for raising dairy cows within major cities like New York and Chicago in the mid-1800s that led to the sanitation problems that contaminated milk with tuberculosis and typhoid, sickening and killing many thousands of children. This tragedy led to the first mandatory pasteurization in a number of large cities in the early 1900s, which gradually evolved into the near-universal pasteurization that exists today, despite concerns expressed over the years that raw milk is nutritionally much more beneficial than the pasteurized variety.

It was modern-day versions of such feedlots that may well have given us the scourge of *E. coli* O157:H7 during the early 1980s. This mutation of normally harmless *E. coli* bacteria is a major player in the battles that have developed over raw milk in the last few years, as you'll see in several of the stories of sick children that are prominent in this book.

Even though *E. coli* O157:H7 likely grew out of factory-farming practices, the fact that it can contaminate raw milk has been a major factor in calls by public health officials to ban raw milk entirely. That irony prompted one individual who comments frequently on my blog, Dave Milano, to observe:

> There are two distinctly different schools of thought at work here. One trusts and welcomes industrialization and centralization; the other is suspicious of it. A philosophical Grand Canyon sits between.
>
> To those with no apprehension about centralized, production-oriented food systems, raw milk will always be a dangerous intruder, discussed only in terms of its relative safety for this or that individual. Raw milk supporters, on the other hand, see a much broader, and I would say much more instructive, picture, that considers overall public health, or more properly, the overall healthfulness of a population.[5]

2. Holistic Health Care Versus Conventional Health Care

Acupuncturists and naturopaths work in different worlds than internists and ear-nose-and-throat specialists. The alternative practitioners are focused on energy fields and total body functioning, while the conventional practitioners are focused on individual organs and germs. Now, admittedly, there have been some interesting efforts to bring these two worlds together, via integrated health centers (my internist is part of one, and she encourages me to meditate to reduce my stress), but these remain fairly isolated.

The one place where these worlds are clashing on an increasingly regular basis is in the arena of public health, over the issues of bacteria and raw milk. Because public health professionals tend to come from the conventional health world, they see bacteria as threats to public health.

The holistic universe tends to focus on "good" bacteria, such as those in yogurt and probiotic nutritional supplements. In this view, good bacteria help battle bad bacteria that enter our bodies, reducing our chances of becoming ill from pathogens such as *E. coli* O157:H7. Moreover, the growing concerns over so-called super-bugs like MRSA (methicillin-resistant *Staphylococcus aureus*) are prompting efforts to increase sanitation of our environment and, in the view of holistic practitioners, simply worsening such problems as food allergies in children.

Increasingly, these different views have clashed over the question of whether raw milk produced under sanitary conditions is a public health hazard. For conventionally trained public health professionals, who see dangerous bacteria around every corner, the growing popularity of raw milk does indeed present a growing public health hazard. Yet consumers of raw milk know that their farmers apply a number of techniques to significantly reduce any such risks.

3. Food Rights Versus Consumer Protection

For most of this country's history, there was no real tension in this conflict, since food rights took precedence, much as individual rights have taken precedence since the founding of the republic. Even as cities like New York and Chicago mandated pasteurization, they still allowed for the availability of so-called certified raw milk—unpasteurized milk produced by inspected dairies under highly sanitary conditions. But beginning in 1947, when Michigan became the first state in the nation to mandate pasteurization of all milk, and nearly half the states followed suit, the pendulum has swung increasingly toward the food safety side.

Because the movement has been so gradual, it's easy not to even notice, until you look back in time. As recently as the mid-1980s, raw milk could be shipped across state lines, and the nation's then-largest raw dairy, in California, had eight thousand cows and more than a hundred thousand customers in nine states. The Reagan administration, stressing individual over government rights, resisted calls by a Ralph Nader–backed organization that the FDA impose a ban on the sale or shipment of raw milk across state lines, and eventually had to be coerced to do so by a federal judge.[6, 7]

A little over twenty years later, the nation's currently largest raw dairy, also in California, had fewer than four hundred cows and an estimated thirty-five thousand customers who purchased its milk retail. In 2008, its owner was charged with a felony for shipping raw milk to customers in other states, many of whom had ordered from him in desperation because their states prohibit the sale of unpasteurized milk, even directly from the farm. And this time the US president, Barack Obama, had declared himself in favor of FDA oversight of raw milk even in advance of being elected.[8]

As raw milk has become more difficult to obtain in many areas of the country, committed consumers sometimes travel hours every couple of weeks to obtain the milk they so value. Or sometimes they obtain it, from farmers or vendors who ship it illegally from states where it's allowed into states where it's not. All of which prompted Pete Kennedy, the head of the Farm-to-Consumer Legal Defense Fund—an organization that provides legal help to raw dairy farmers targeted for penalties by state agriculture and public health regulators—to tell a recent conference of dairy regulators: "This is a freedom of choice issue. The sale of raw milk is illegal in half the states. Young mothers are going across state lines to get raw milk. . . . We are making otherwise law-abiding citizens into criminals."

What he might have added is that individual freedom and rights have nearly always taken precedence in this country. A fundamental premise underlies our Bill of Rights and its protections against self incrimination and unreasonable searches of our homes, along with the right to legal representation and trial by jury: that it is preferable to let dozens or hundreds of guilty individuals go free so that we avoid convicting even a single innocent person via questionable measures like arbitrary police home invasions or kangaroo courts. Applying the same logic to food rights, it might be said that consumers should have the right to obtain the foods of their choice, even if in some cases it means assuming some minimal risk of becoming ill.

It's this issue of rights versus protection that is arousing the most serious passion around raw milk and, increasingly, other foods. In recent years, we have seen highly publicized cases of sickness, including some deaths, from food-borne illness carried in such common foods as fresh spinach, peanut butter, hamburger meat, and fast food from Taco Bell. Increasingly fearful consumers demand that the government "protect" us—via more inspectors and tougher penalties on sellers of contaminated products—and the government tries to comply.

Yet the more the government tries to protect us, the worse some of the food and health problems, expressed via exploding rates of chronic disease and the appearance of "superbugs" like MRSA, seem to become. More health and medical authorities are questioning whether the ever-widening use of sanitation techniques, including pasteurization, irradiation, the overuse of antibiotics, and even including sanitizing soaps and wipes, could be eliminating beneficial bacteria that not only keep pathogens at bay but also boost the nutritional value of foods.

So now, in the early twenty-first century, the debate about the role of food as a cause of illness or a determinant of health grows ever louder. As you'll see when you read *The Raw Milk Revolution*, the extent to which the illness or health component takes precedence is key to which side one tends to take in the debate.

If you're like the mothers of two young children I describe who may well have become seriously ill from raw milk in 2006, you tend to focus most heavily on the dangers of illness from foods. If you're like the mothers of other children who have watched their children's allergy symptoms dissipate or seen the frequency of their ear infections decrease after consuming raw milk, well, then your focus is on the health advantages to be gained from certain foods.

In my experience writing about the debate that swirls around raw milk, I've come to realize that, to the extent to which we obsess about germs in raw milk (and other foods), we are less receptive to the idea that nutrient-dense foods help combat or prevent disease. The reverse seems to hold as well: To the extent we become enamored of the health benefits of raw milk, we let go of worries about becoming ill from it and its dangers to public health. We figure that the highly visible benefits will outweigh any small dangers.

So intense are the passions of partisans on both sides of the issue that it's very difficult for many people to achieve a realistic balance. As the struggle over raw milk makes clear, it's nearly impossible to satisfy everyone's concerns about balancing protection with rights.

Muddying the waters even further is the fact that the divisions don't break down nearly as easily into liberal and conservative camps as do other political issues like abortion or gun rights. Some easterners I know who are otherwise liberal are increasingly fearful of food-borne illness and feel raw milk is a terrible danger, while others I know who are completely conservative on issues such as abortion or guns feel the government should steer clear of prohibiting any food, be it raw milk or McDonald's hamburgers. Perhaps because of such political confusion, it's been difficult to organize consumers either pro or con on the issue of food rights (though such efforts are definitely under way, most notably through the National Independent Consumers and Farmers Association, and its affiliates, in more than fifteen states).[9]

In spite of, or because of, the strong feelings and political confusion, our country has moved ever more forcefully toward the protection side of the equation. *The Raw Milk Revolution* questions the wisdom of that tilt.

CHAPTER ONE

Why Is the Government Kicking Around a Bunch of Small-Time Dairy Farmers?

Back in early 2006, though I was well into my fifties and regularly wrote about health, I knew nothing about raw milk. I just assumed all milk was pasteurized. Actually, I hadn't thought much about milk since my growing-up years and twenties, when I drank up to a quart a day. Like many baby boomers, I had forsaken dairy products in general as part of a drive to keep my weight and cholesterol in check.

Then one day in February or March, while perusing the US Food and Drug Administration's Web site,[1] I saw an item from the previous December that eight people had become ill from drinking unpasteurized milk at a place called Dee Creek Farm in Washington State, and that the farm was prohibited from selling products. Its Web site[2] showed pretty pictures of cows, children, and adults in a farm setting. The idea of people drinking unpasteurized milk, though completely foreign to me, seemed strangely exotic. Wasn't this the stuff that caused mass epidemics during the 1800s, until we were saved by Louis Pasteur's simple process of heating milk to 161 degrees for fifteen to twenty seconds? Could this be another example of a food with powerful nutritional properties that had gone unrecognized in our modern society, much like oatmeal, fish, and broccoli, which had come into fashion in the 1980s and 1990s? Not to mention the more recent interest in less processed foods, as evidenced by the hugely popular bulk bins at Whole Foods Market, filled with raw lentils, nuts, and beans of all descriptions.

I was in the midst of a career shift at the time, moving from being a part-time entrepreneur and writer specializing in small business to being a writer specializing in health care. I had become increasingly interested in, and captivated by, alternative health approaches, both personally (more on that later) and as a writer. For several years, I had written a column on small business for BusinessWeek.com, and as part of my career shift I wanted to write more about the business of health.

I had found the FDA site to be an excellent repository of information. As an advocate of entrepreneurship and small business, I often felt the agency aggressively singled out for enforcement producers or products associated with alternative health, which tended to be smaller companies. An item about an FDA "warning letter" (a possible prelude to serious legal action) to several small producers of cherry juice in Michigan for supposedly making unwarranted health claims led me in June 2006 to write a column[3] suggesting the agency was coming down unnecessarily hard on small orchards producing a wholesome, healthy product. Their health claims seemed tamer than those by major corporations, such as Kellogg's claims that its HeartSmart cereal is "the best way to treat heart disease," and Welch's, which suggested grape juice can inhibit breast cancer tumor formation, act as an "anti-aging" food, and "may have a positive effect on blood pressure." Yet neither of these corporations had encountered FDA opposition.

In any event, I tried calling Dee Creek to get its side of the story, but couldn't get beyond the answering machine. I figured the owners were rightfully nervous and didn't want to draw more attention to themselves by speaking with a reporter. From a reporter's perspective, I had called too late. In my experience, you have to reach individuals accused by the government of wrongdoing very quickly to learn the details of their situation—before they hire lawyers who advise the accused not to speak to the media.

So I waited for what I guessed would be another instance of problems with raw milk. To keep up on happenings, I entered the term "raw milk" into Google Alerts, which e-mailed me each time the term showed up in an article or on a blog.

That summer, I spent most of my weekends in western New Hampshire, at a small vacation condo, about midway between Lake Sunapee and Hanover, the home of Dartmouth College. On Saturday mornings, my wife and I generally drove to a wonderful Vermont farmer's market featuring fresh veggies, cheeses, and crafts.

One Saturday in July, I noticed a stand at the market with a hand-lettered wooden sign: RAW MILK. I introduced myself to Kathy, the farmer selling the milk. She looked to be in her midfifties, and definitely had the farmer appearance with big coveralls and a checked shirt. I asked her about her milk. How long had she been in the raw milk business? What did she feed her cows? Did she use antibiotics? I had gotten my questions from hunting around the Internet and reading a few of the many pro-raw-milk sites.

Kathy was very friendly and patient, telling me her four cows were "raised with love" and nearly entirely pasture-fed—grazing outdoors in the summer and eating hay in the winter. She avoided antibiotics unless the cows were diagnosed with a disease that would otherwise kill them.

I decided she was trustworthy, especially with the way she answered the antibiotics question, and I bought a gallon, for $3. That Saturday, I had my first glass of raw milk at lunch, with a homemade chocolate chip cookie I also purchased at the market. Suddenly I was back in my childhood, with my all-time favorite snack. The milk was as creamy and rich tasting as it looked, with a slight sweetness I didn't recall from my childhood milk.

But I'd be lying if I didn't admit that overhanging the experience was an anxiety-laden question provoked by my American history classes highlighting the importance of pasteurization in saving lives: Might this wonderful milk kill me? I actually went to sleep wondering whether I'd wake up.

I later learned from other raw milk drinkers that this initial concern is fairly common. I'm still not sure I understand the psychological dynamics whereby I could bring myself to ingest a drink that my upbringing had taught me could kill me. I suspect that countering that information was the knowledge that lots of people were doing it, and I wasn't reading about people dropping dead. Maybe it was a little like jumping off garage roofs or having paper clip fights as a kid—you were told about the terrible dangers, but didn't believe they would happen to you.

Of course, there was no bad reaction of any sort, and I became a regular customer, hauling my cooler with chemical ice to the market each Saturday, to keep my milk cold. I came to learn from Kathy that she usually had three cows producing milk at any one time, and that she tried to provide regular customers like me with milk from her Guernsey, Selena. Kathy felt that Guernseys produce milk with the highest beta-carotene content. Besides, she thought Selena's milk tasted best. Nora was her second favorite. (I would eventually learn that there are wide differences of opinion among dairy farmers and raw milk aficionados about the relative advantages of milk from Guernseys, Jerseys, Holsteins, and Ayrshires; some like Jerseys for their especially high butterfat content, while others prefer Holsteins or Ayrshires for their taste.) I loved the fact that the cow providing my milk could even be identified, given that the average container of pasteurized milk contains the output of perhaps hundreds of unidentifiable cows.

Just as important to me was that, now, when I finally wrote about raw milk, I couldn't be accused of being a hypocrite.

On the morning of September 26, I received a news item from an alternative medicine site, www.mercola.com, about a dairy that had been shut down in California because four children had become ill from raw milk that was said to contain *E. coli* O157:H7, a pathogenic variety of the *E. coli* bacteria, which isn't usually harmful. At the same time, the United States was in the midst of a scare over raw spinach from California. In communities around the country, children and adults alike were falling ill with severe diarrhea from the same pathogen, *E. coli* O157:H7.

Each day, the numbers increased—100, 125, 160. Some people became so sick they had to be put on kidney dialysis, and two actually died. Public health authorities were pretty sure the contaminated raw spinach came from California, but they seemed powerless to isolate the source, and could do nothing except recommend that supermarkets remove raw spinach from their shelves.

I did some quick research on the dairy, Organic Pastures Dairy Co. of Fresno. Like Dee Creek, its Web site[4] featured pretty photos of calves, children, and cows being milked, along with a family photo of about a dozen men, women, and teens who apparently ran the farm.

From the FDA I learned that, a year earlier, the agency had sent Organic Pastures' owner, Mark McAfee, a warning letter ordering the dairy to discontinue shipping raw milk to customers outside California, since such shipments were a violation of federal prohibitions on raw milk in interstate commerce.

I quickly telephoned McAfee and, surprisingly, got right through to him. He had been silent for nearly two weeks, he told me, ever since officials of California's Department of Food and Agriculture first informed him of the children's illnesses and slapped a quarantine on his dairy, meaning that no food-related items could be shipped to or from it. He expected that any day the state and federal inspectors who had been roaming his three-hundred-cow dairy—without finding any evidence of *E. coli* O157:H7—would do what they'd promised and pack up and go home. Each day, though, they seemed to have another demand—a new crate of plastic bottles to open, another piece of equipment or machinery to haul out for examination—that kept them inspecting and McAfee making changes in how he stored his supplies and arranged his milking.

On this morning, he decided, there would be no more Mister Nice Guy. And since I was the first media person to call following his decision, he would speak with me.

"This is a full assault against us," he told me, speaking forcefully, in machine-gun fashion. "It's a war against raw milk. . . . They've done hundreds and hundreds of tests and found zero pathogens." If the authorities didn't back off and allow him to reopen, "We're going to sue them for $100 million."

As I would come to know over the ensuing months, Mark McAfee didn't mince his words, nor did he shirk from standing up to government regulators.

He described for me a situation in which a dozen or more guys in white coveralls and plastic gloves from the CDFA and the FDA were combing every crevice and corner of his dairy, taking milk and manure samples from cows, inspecting his bulk tanks, tearing apart packaging, and digging up soil samples. He said he had voluntarily followed up the quarantine order by recalling his milk from the shelves of Whole Foods and other health store outlets.

He also told me that he had once been a paramedic, and thus knew a lot about health and disease. Over the previous six years, he and his wife, daughter, son, and son-in-law had grown the dairy to the point that it supplied more than thirty thousand customers with raw milk each day, representing nearly 90 percent of the California raw milk market. These people were now deprived of their raw milk, and he was getting hundreds of e-mails from upset customers.

What about the children who were sick, I inquired. He told me there seemed to be at least four children who had consumed raw milk and were now ill. (The official number allegedly sickened would eventually grow to six children.) Three had been diagnosed with *E. coli* O157:H7, and one had shigella, a bacterial infection that sometimes occurs when food poisoning is treated with antibiotics. The *E. coli* O157:H7 in the three seemed to be of a different variety than the one plaguing spinach. He said he had visited the two children who were hospitalized, and was told they might have eaten raw spinach; so, in his view, it was possible their *E. coli* came from spinach as well—perhaps a second outbreak. One thing he was sure of, he told me, was that no *E. coli* O157:H7 had been found in any of his cows.

I called the CDFA, and officials there confirmed that nothing had been found in his animals or around his farm. But that didn't mean the bad *E. coli* hadn't come from his dairy's milk, a spokesperson told me: There was "epidemiological evidence" that the children had become sick from raw milk, based on the fact that three of them had the same strain of bad *E. coli,* which was different from the strain in the tainted spinach, and all had drunk raw milk.

I wrote a column about Mark McAfee titled "Getting a Raw Deal?"[5] In it, I described how he felt the officials were unfairly treating him by keeping him shut down, while spinach producers under scrutiny for sending pathogens into the marketplace with their product were allowed to keep operating.

I continued to write about McAfee's situation on my blog[6]—about the tedious process of gaining full approval to actually go back on the market during the first week of October. It turned out the original lifting of the quarantine only covered butter and cheese, not the milk that made up 70 percent of his business. His milk needed to pass tests for somatic cell count—somatic cells being white blood cells that affect the taste and shelf life of the milk; they're considered by some dairy experts to be an indicator of milk cleanliness but don't in themselves make people sick. His count was high, according to readings from the Fresno County Health Department, but within normal ranges according to readings from the California Dairy Herd Improvement Association, Mark reported. And once he reached the normal range in the county test, he had to do it again, since regulations required two normal readings, not one.

This wouldn't be the first time that the "official" readings of raw milk would come back differently from readings done by an outside agency. In this case, Mark attributed the discrepancy to differences in testing equipment—the DHIA used highly sophisticated and carefully calibrated equipment to do its testing, versus the county's manual microscope approach. When I asked a county health official about the discrepancy, he would say only, "Our test is the official test."

Finally, on Friday, October 8, McAfee had full clearance to sell milk. Yet within twenty-four hours, there was another problem. That Saturday, at the Santa Monica Farmer's Market near Los Angeles, three Los Angeles County health inspectors showed up to question the dairy employees running the Organic Pastures stand. The dairy sells raw milk at farmer's markets around the state, typically selling a thousand gallons at each.

After a couple hours of back-and-forth between the health inspectors and the dairy reps, the Organic Pastures people produced the reinstatement documents from California officials, and the inspectors backed off. But not before the inspectors seized several gallons of unlabeled milk used by one of the Organic Pastures reps to demonstrate cheese production, and also not before at least one consumer tried vociferously to convince the health inspectors to find more legitimate targets.

The following week, I telephoned the Los Angeles County Department of Public Health and spoke with Terrance Powell, the director of food inspection, who explained to me that Organic Pastures hadn't shown up for a scheduled hearing that week to explain why it had fifteen to twenty unlabeled bottles of raw milk in its inventory at the Santa Monica Farmer's Market that Saturday, as well as at another farmer's market a few weeks previous.

"There were two complaints . . . about raw milk being sold without labels. . . . Our inspectors investigated and found raw milk being sold without labels."

If Organic Pastures couldn't come up with "mitigating" information, Powell said, the LA department might seek criminal misdemeanor charges against its officials and/or the dairy itself. "I would be willing to" request such charges, he stated. "I would be failing my fiduciary duty if I didn't follow through."

When I sought comment from Mark to the food inspection director's threats, he didn't seem especially concerned. He said his lawyer had recommended skipping the hearing because the complaints were "baseless."

What a crazy way to run a business, I remember thinking, if every Tuesday and Saturday you're being hit with regulatory challenges. Never mind the production interruptions and the stress—what about the impact on customers? Wouldn't they be scared off? I had always assumed that the worst thing to befall a food producer was government charges of health problems.

Just the opposite, as it happens. McAfee said he had received three thousand e-mails during the shutdown from unhappy customers wondering when their raw milk would return. He supplied me with a dozen or so examples from customers thrilled to have their raw milk back.

"It has been a wonderful day here, enjoying our pure, healthy, live milk!" one customer wrote. "My oldest was especially grateful, as after four days of organic pasteurized milk . . . The first thing we did when we got home from picking up our order from the buyer's club was open a beautiful carton of fresh whole milk and drink big glasses of it. I actually considered picking up a disposable camera and taking pictures of us enjoying the milk and sending them to you! (We don't have a digital.) Then I made a wonderful smoothie with the kefir and this afternoon we had popcorn with delicious raw butter all over it."

Another customer said simply: "Just to let you know that yesterday we bought your milk again at Henry's in La Mesa. Yippee!"

Even more convincing was the fact that once Organic Pastures' milk came back on the market, business shot up close to 10 percent. McAfee said he had come to view the events of late September and early October as "a perfect marketing storm"—that is, the dairy's exoneration by regulators together with huge amounts of publicity, all helping feed what he calls "the raw foods revolution."

As for the threatened criminal charges from the LA health authorities, McAfee told me the problems just "went away." I tried reaching Powell at least four times to get his version of what happened, but he never returned any of my calls.

Strange world, this world of raw milk.

Nearly before I could catch my breath, in mid-October another curious situation involving raw milk came to my attention. An Ann Arbor, Michigan, paper, the *Ann Arbor News* (which has since closed down), published a brief article about a farmer, Richard Hebron, who had been nabbed in a "sting" operation delivering raw milk to customers in the university town.

Within minutes of receiving the item, I found Hebron's number and telephoned him. He picked up the phone, and confirmed that, yes, he had been forced off the road by the Michigan State Police a few days earlier. "They treated me little better than a drug dealer," he said. He was much more soft-spoken than Mark McAfee as he spilled out his disturbing story.

On the morning of October 13, as Hebron was cruising down Interstate 94 in his small pickup truck on his way into Ann Arbor, a Michigan State Police cruiser signaled him over and ordered him to get out and put his hands on the hood. The trooper patted him down and directed him to drive a mile up the road to a rest area. There four or five Michigan Department of Agriculture agents showed him a search warrant, took his wallet and cell phone, and began off-loading some of the 453 gallons of fresh raw milk he carried in coolers, along with kefir and butter made from raw milk—some $7,000 worth of product.

When the agents realized they didn't have enough space in their cars to take all the food, they gave Hebron a choice. He could drive the truck seventy miles to the state capital of Lansing, where the MDA is headquartered, and the agents would complete their off-loading. Or they would seize the truck, and he could find his way home from the roadside. Some choice. Hebron drove his truck to Lansing. They wouldn't even let him telephone his wife and let her know what had happened.

They had a reason for not wanting Hebron to contact his wife. That's because, as Hebron was being detained, one agent was telephoning a colleague and giving the go-ahead for the next part of the sting operation. In Vandalia, 140 miles to the west, MDA and state police agents knocked on the front door of the Hebrons' tiny house and greeted his wife, Annette, with a search warrant. Over the next three hours, five agents rummaged through the Hebrons' business and personal papers, including things like bank statements, medical information, and grocery receipts. They confiscated Richard Hebron's business files and computer. They debated about whether to take the couple's answering machine and telephone, and finally decided these wouldn't yield any "evidence." They even went through the family's refrigerator, discussing whether a frozen chicken in the freezer was possibly "intended for sale" and thus evidence. (They decided it wasn't, and left it.)

All the while, co-op members were phoning in, wondering where their milk, kefir, and eggs were. Annette explained the delay, and finally told one of the agents, "You don't know how many people you are making angry." He rolled his eyes, as if to say, *Whoop-dee-do.*

Simultaneously, agents executed a third search warrant, on Morgan & York, the Ann Arbor gourmet food store where Richard distributed the raw milk and other dairy and meat products to more than two hundred co-op members.

I telephoned Katherine Fedder, the director of the MDA's Food and Dairy Division, who told me the "sting" had been planned for six months—that it was triggered by reports from public health authorities of several members of a family becoming ill from raw milk the previous spring. Privacy laws prevented her or the local department of public health, which had investigated, from telling me who the family was.

Without their confiscated computer, the Hebrons were off the Internet, and so couldn't communicate via e-mail. I mailed Richard a copy of my BusinessWeek.com column[7] via the US Postal Service.

While many individuals might have been prepared to run out and purchase another computer, the Hebrons weren't that well off financially. Richard had dreamed of becoming a farmer ever since he was in high school. After graduation, he worked for a number of years as a cabinetmaker. Finally, seventeen years previously, he'd saved up enough money to make a down payment on some farmland in Vandalia. He owned forty acres, but still had to lease seventy acres to give him the grazing land he needed. The Hebrons lived in a tiny three-room house with their two children.

Needless to say, Richard Hebron's co-op members in Ann Arbor, and in nearby Detroit, where he also distributed products, didn't receive their orders that week, or the week after, for that matter. In my column and on my blog, dozens of co-op members expressed their outrage over what some referred to as the MDA's "Gestapo tactics" in confiscating products and conducting search warrants of a home and business.

But the matter didn't end with that Friday's three-pronged assault on Hebron's truck, his home, and the Morgan & York store. A few days later, the MDA was back at Morgan & York. MDA inspector Beth Howell—"Inspector Beth" as she was known to co-owner Tommy York—walked in with a five-paragraph cease-and-desist order and told York to sign it. While the technical language ordered the store "to cease and desist in the delivery, holding, or offering for sale of adulterated or misbranded food," the real purpose was to prevent the store from allowing the cooperative to distribute its products from the store's storage area, as it had done for the previous two years.

Tommy York didn't hesitate to obey the order, knowing that if he didn't, he would likely lose his MDA-regulated food license. "I'm wise enough to know when to sign," the gregarious York told me. Food accounted for about one-third of the store's $3 million annual sales and, equally important, it was growing at a rate of 10 percent annually and provided higher margins than his wine and liquor sales, which were flat.

York had offered his store's rear storage area as a distribution outlet for the co-op at no charge because, as he said, "We were trying to be enlightened good neighbors." He figured that if a couple of hundred people who obviously were committed to consuming high-quality food came to his store for co-op pickups each week, "Maybe they'll come over and buy from us." And they did.

But reality was reality. "I have to toe the line or I lose my livelihood . . . I'll never get my father paid back"—on the loan York's father and some of his friends had made for Tommy and his partner to buy the store in 2001. How much was that loan? "I don't even want to say," he told me with a sigh.

"As a citizen, I want to fight, but as a businessman, I can't," York explained. He felt especially let down by the regulators, with whom he was accustomed to having a friendly professional relationship. "I want the Agriculture Department to help me. Their tactics are so heavy-handed. They could have just rang us up and told us they wanted to meet with us. They could have said, 'We have some concerns,' and we could make some adjustments in how this is handled. This whole sting thing is ridiculous."

But there was more. Because Richard Hebron obtained the unpasteurized milk for the Family Farms Cooperative from a farm just over the border from Michigan, in Indiana, the MDA had alerted the US Food and Drug Administration, which enforces a federal ban on interstate shipments of raw milk for consumption.

Within a few days of the raid, two FDA agents visited the dairy owned by David Hochstetler, an Amish farmer, and inquired about his relationship with Hebron. I didn't speak with David until a few months later. Because of his worry about the investigation, he asked Richard Hebron to keep his name out of the articles on the sting. When Richard asked me to cooperate, I agreed, and didn't follow up directly with Hochstetler. It would have been difficult in any event—he didn't have a telephone, let alone a computer.

Just when I thought things couldn't get any worse on the raw milk front, I learned, as Thanksgiving 2006 approached, of another dairy farm in trouble with the law. A tiny news item in an Ohio newspaper reported that a Kentucky dairy farmer had been fined $500 by an Ohio municipal court for illegally selling raw milk in the state.[8] Because the item was so brief and the fine so tiny, I wanted to assume the case was simple and inconsequential as well. I debated with myself about whether to try to reach the farmer, Gary Oaks. But I had seen enough "small stories" turn out to be significant that I called him up.

Gary's wife, Dawn, answered the phone and told me that, though the case had actually occurred eight months earlier, the previous March, it was probably good I was calling this particular evening. The couple hadn't wanted to talk about the case while it was still unresolved, but now that it was settled, and Gary was feeling better, well, maybe this was the time to finally go public with what happened.

Gary feeling better . . . what was that about?

An hour later, Oaks called me back and began telling me his story. He was forty-three, he said, and Dawn thirty-nine, and two years earlier they had chucked conventional careers in inventory management (for him) and health care (for her), to purchase the tiny Double O Farm in northern Kentucky, about forty-five minutes south of Cincinnati, along with a herd of ten cows. One of the first things they did was establish a herd-share program, since the sale of raw milk is illegal in Ohio and Kentucky (and twenty-one other states). A herd share, sometimes referred to as a cow-share, essentially gives participants partial ownership of a dairy's herd, and therefore its milk, for payment of a share price and ongoing payments for herd feed and lodging.

For Gary and Dawn, the shareholder arrangement enabled them to fulfill their personal desire to make milk available to consumers in what they believed was a healthier form. It also enabled them to escape the mass-production-commodity cycle that had seen an estimated fifteen hundred Kentucky dairies bite the dust in the decade between 1993 and 2003 alone.

The herd-share arrangement was a quick success. Word spread so rapidly that within a few months, 160 Cincinnati-area families had signed up, paying $75 a share and $25 a month for herd maintenance, which entitled them to a gallon of milk each week. Many bought two or three shares. Gary delivered to various drop-off points in the Cincinnati area as a convenience to the shareholders.

For nearly a year and a half, everything went as planned. Oaks made his weekly deliveries, and the shareholders were thrilled to have a regular supply of raw milk.

But on March 6, everything changed. At about 1:15 that afternoon, Oaks arrived at a Cincinnati parking lot that serves a school and a church, for what he thought would be a routine drop-off. He got out of his truck, opened the trailer, and began handing out bottles of milk to a few of the dozen or so shareholders present. At this point, his recollection of what happened became hazy.

I later called a few shareholders who were there and had witnessed the ensuing events to try to fill in the entire story. Joanne Miller, of Morrow, Ohio, remembered vividly what happened next. "I was placing empty bottles in carriers when I noticed a Cincinnati police cruiser moving through the parking lot slowly toward the trailer. Another cruiser followed. . . . Officers moved toward the herd-share owners and told them not to pick up the milk that had already been set out and actually moved in to prevent members from picking up the milk."

Out of several unmarked cars emerged non-uniformed men who "gathered near the tailgate of the trailer." Only one would identify himself, an agent of the Ohio Department of Agriculture, Joanne said. Other agents were there from the Kentucky Department of Public Health and the US Food and Drug Administration. Joanne estimated there were about eight agents there, plus the four Cincinnati police officers. As the agents began confiscating the milk both from the truck and from a few shareholders, and loading it into an ODA van, the agents told objecting shareholders, "What is happening here is not your concern."

This upset the shareholders, who began shouting that the milk belonged to them, that the agents had no right to it. One of the shareholders stood on the truck trailer's tailgate and waved her shareholder documents at the agents, who ignored her.

Sensing that the situation might be getting out of hand, the Cincinnati cops called for reinforcements, and two additional cruisers arrived. In the meantime, several plainclothes agents moved to separate Oaks from his shareholders. The confrontation with police was immediately upsetting to Oaks, a soft-spoken man who grew up on a Mississippi farm and had only once in his life even been stopped for speeding. At this point, it all became a terrifying blur for him.

As Oaks recalls it, they moved him toward one of the unmarked cars and ordered him in. "They asked me what I was doing. One said, 'You're in a lot of trouble. You've broken all kinds of laws.'"

Oaks didn't know what to say. "I was ignorant. I didn't know it was illegal to drink milk. I hate to sound ignorant."

Then they moved him from that car into a second car, and the routine started over again, except more intensively. One agent was shouting from the back, and another in the front was demanding that he write something that sounded to him like a confession that he was selling unpasteurized milk. He began feeling ill. "They were telling me what to write, that I wouldn't sell milk." He started to write something, but can't remember what.

(The ODA later produced a "Witness Statement" in response to my request, with block printing, signed by Oaks and an ODA investigator: "We run a cow-share business in Kentucky. Sell shares of cows to people for $75 a share . . ." It included a few more details about the maintenance fee and delivery schedule and concluded, "Whole milk is not pasteurized.")

When Oaks emerged from the car, several shareholders said he looked terrible and asked the officers to call 911. "We are 911," one of the officers stated. A shareholder decided to call 911 on her cell phone, seeking an ambulance. The agents moved Oaks into a third car. He told them he was feeling awful, got out of the car, and slumped to the ground. An ambulance arrived and took him to a hospital. His blood pressure had soared to more than 200/156. "They were shocked I wasn't dead," Gary told me. He was released later that day, apparently not having suffered a heart attack.

An ODA spokesperson wouldn't admit they had gone too far, telling me, "Our officials questioned Mr. Oaks, as did federal officials. They were trying to learn about what he was doing, what the substance was, and why it was being brought into Ohio."

Oaks continued to feel ill over the next few days. He had nightmares of "police and agents coming out from behind bushes and buildings." He couldn't milk the cows. A few days later, the feelings worsened. "I was choking, I couldn't get my breath." Dawn took him back to the hospital, and this time he was admitted for several days.

The one piece of good news was that his shareholders had sprung into action. More than a hundred met within days at a local church and tried to figure out how they could help the farm and the Oakses. The most immediate issue was the cows these shareholders owned—they needed to be milked twice a day, and most of the city-folk shareholders knew little about the process beyond the fact that their milk arrived in bottles every week. And because their cows were Jerseys, they were sensitive to who milked them, preferring consistent milkers.

Fortunately, three shareholders who lived close to the Double O Farm had also been farmers, and at one of several meetings the shareholders held, these individuals volunteered to do the milking. The next pressing issue was how to get the milk bottled and out to the shareholders, since Oaks couldn't deliver.

Here another shareholder, Kimberly Gelhaus of Cincinnati, dove in. "I took over coordinating carpooling. . . . We had to coordinate deliveries for 160 families." Several dozen shareholders became involved in shuttling milk from the farm to shareholders in Kentucky and Ohio, some driving several hours each way. Others handled bottling, and still more volunteered to gather hay and do yard work around the farm, or bring food to Dawn and her three children, all under age ten.

As the winter wore on, Oaks would be hospitalized twice more. Doctors concluded he was suffering from post-traumatic stress syndrome, a stress disorder most common among combat soldiers. A couple of shareholders with psychology backgrounds provided counseling.

Adding to the Oakses' stress was that they didn't have health insurance. By the end of spring, Gary's medical bills were approaching $50,000. And then there was the matter of his legal problems—from Kentucky, Ohio, and the federal government. As things turned out, Kentucky officials backed off from filing formal charges after an informal hearing by the Kentucky

Milk Safety Board. But Ohio eventually filed charges accusing Oaks of illegally selling raw milk and an unlabeled product. His legal bills soared past $10,000.

By the summer, life finally began improving. Oaks was feeling well enough to work on the farm. He was able to negotiate a reduction in his medical bills with the hospitals. Shareholders passed the hat to take care of his legal bills. Two shareholders even agreed to loan him funds to move the farm to a badly needed larger tract of land half an hour from his existing farm.

On November 2, he went to a county municipal court in Reynoldsburg, Ohio, and pleaded no contest to violating Ohio's dairy licensing and labeling laws. He was fined $415, along with an additional $85 in court costs. The FDA also sent him a warning letter against interstate sales of raw milk.

Kimberly and other shareholders continued to carpool to get milk delivered to shareholders, since Oaks didn't want to challenge the FDA's prohibition about crossing state lines to make deliveries in Ohio.

What was it that got the state and federal officials so aggressively on Oaks' tail? No officials ever even suggested anyone became ill from his milk. Rather, the immediate culprit appears to have been a disgruntled neighbor who didn't like the mooing of Oaks' cows. The neighbor had called local officials in the past, but they had begged off because the Double O Farm was zoned for farming. He had apparently then resorted to complaining to state agriculture officials about Oaks' raw milk distribution, and they were only too happy to take the bait.

When I spoke to officials at the Ohio Department of Agriculture, they said that Oaks was just one piece of a much bigger problem. Early in 2006, a young boy and an elderly man in the Dayton area had become seriously ill from campylobacter, a pathogen that is a source of food-borne illness, in raw milk. The ODA had gone after at least three other dairies selling raw milk in the state, and suspected that the bad milk came from a dairy owed by Carol Schmitmeyer, who with her husband and five children operated a three-hundred-acre farm in Versailles, Ohio.

In late 2005, she established a herd-sharing arrangement to make raw milk available to about 150 people in the Dayton area who were eager for the product. The lawyer who drew up the papers had previously worked for the ODA, she told me, and thus she assumed the arrangement would pass muster with the agency.

In September 2006—right around the times of the crackdowns in California and Michigan—the ODA demanded in a hearing that Carol's dairy license be revoked. The hearing examiner, who was an outsider hired by the agriculture agency, agreed, declaring that the herd-sharing agreements were "a thinly veiled attempt to evade the prohibitions against selling raw milk" in Ohio, and ordered her license be revoked.

Revoking a Grade A dairy license is a serious financial threat to any dairy farm, since it removes a significant source of income. Schmitmeyer decided to appeal the decision to state court. "If they take our license away, we lose the farm," she told me that November.

At this point, I felt badly for the farmers—ordinary, hardworking people. But I wondered: What about the children who had been made sick by the raw milk? If raw milk made children ill, shouldn't there be a penalty? Don't we deserve such protection from our government?

CHAPTER TWO

Raw Milk and the Upside-Down World of Food-Borne Illness

As I discussed in the previous chapter, milk, as in pasteurized milk, was something I took for granted through much of my life, since I didn't know there was an alternative. I suspect the situation was pretty much the same for milk-drinking Americans through much of the 1800s with regard to unpasteurized milk, because that's all there was.

From all we can tell, unpasteurized milk, whether from a cow or goat or camel, was overall a fine product, extolled in the Bible (as in "the land of milk and honey") and prescribed by physicians of the ages to help cure all manner of diseases. I have a book first published in 1905 called *Milk Diet: As a Remedy for Chronic Disease,*[1] written by a medical doctor, that collects much of the knowledge about raw milk until that time; it recommends raw milk as a cure for everything from asthma to rheumatism to high blood pressure.

Raw milk began attracting attention in the 1840s. This interest continued through much of the rest of that century as the United States experienced the Industrial Revolution, with millions of people moving from the countryside to the cities in search of improved wages and lifestyles. It's not unlike what's been happening in China in recent years.

To bring milk supplies closer to population centers, cows were moved into cities as well. But people at that time had little understanding about the importance of sanitation and refrigeration, and milk became a breeding ground for diseases: tuberculosis, typhoid fever, diphtheria, and severe streptococcal infections. It was in this context that Louis Pasteur developed his process for heating foods (he actually started with wine) for brief periods to kill pathogens. When milk was heated to 161 degrees Fahrenheit for fifteen to twenty seconds, it stopped being a breeding ground for such diseases.

In the late 1800s and early 1900s, pasteurization was seen as a miracle of sorts. The rate of childhood deaths in cities like Philadelphia and Boston plunged from 50 percent in the 1840s to less than 10 percent. Nationally, some 25 percent of all food-borne illness was caused by raw milk as late as the 1930s, according to officials at the US Centers for Disease Control (CDC).

One paradox of the government's implicit 2006 declaration of war on raw milk that I described in the previous chapter is that the diseases that gave raw milk such a historical black eye—tuberculosis, typhoid fever, and diphtheria—have pretty much been eradicated. Those were communicable diseases, and thus could be spread not only by food and water but in some cases by human contact as well. Once the disease was planted in a few people, it would be spread via mini epidemics, sometimes as quickly as from any food.

These diseases were slowed considerably during the early 1900s—likely as much or more by modern sewerage systems and improvements in sanitation throughout the food system as by pasteurization. New vaccines discovered in the late 1800s and early 1900s eventually put the finishing touches on typhoid fever and diphtheria, in particular.

The public health problems that upset the authorities in Michigan, California, and Ohio beginning in 2006 had nothing to do with the diseases that led to pasteurization in the 1800s. Rather, the new problems were exclusively food-borne diseases—illnesses caused by pathogens such as *E. coli* O157:H7 and campylobacter. These diseases are spread primarily by food and water—it's very difficult to catch them from other people. Indeed, it's not unusual for one or two members of a family to become ill from one of these pathogens, while others do not experience any symptoms.

Here is how a scientist with the CDC explained the situation in a recent scientific paper:[2] "Fear of contracting typhoid fever from watered milk . . . [is] now part of the distant past. . . . Nonetheless, at the beginning of the 21st century, food-borne disease remains a major threat to public health, as new pathogens and products have emerged."

The most notable example is *E. coli* O157:H7, which was first discovered in 1982 during an outbreak of food poisoning affecting forty-seven people in Michigan and Oregon. The pathogen's launching pad was thought to be hamburger patties that originated in Michigan. *E. coli* O157:H7 has since been implicated in many of the most notorious outbreaks of food-borne illness, including about three hundred raw spinach illnesses in September and October 2006 that coincided with the illnesses of six children associated with raw milk in California.[3]

Why did *E. coli* O157:H7 not make an appearance until the 1980s? That's something I'll examine in a later chapter, but suffice it to say that while no one knows for sure, a number of scientists have speculated that it is the result of overuse of antibiotics to control disease in livestock crowded into massive feedlots, as well as overly heavy feeding of grains rather than grass and hay to cattle, which have combined to stimulate newly dangerous pathogen variants—"super-bugs," according to some.

While the highly feared *E. coli* O157:H7 occasionally makes people very sick, as you'll see later in this chapter, it generally doesn't hold a candle to the communicable diseases of the 1800s in terms of virulence. Those were highly dangerous illnesses, generally killing large percentages of the people stricken. The food-borne illnesses of the late twentieth and early twenty-first centuries are very mild by comparison. Most often, victims experience several days of vomiting or diarrhea, never visit a hospital, and then recover and resume their normal activities. Those individuals at greatest risk of complications are mostly pregnant women, young children, and the elderly.

Most of the information I'm providing here about illnesses carried by raw milk and other foods is based on what I've read on the CDC Web site, in CDC scientific papers, and in various science journals. But how do outbreaks play out in real life? How are they tracked? What are the experiences of people who become ill, in terms of not only their symptoms but also determining what made them ill, dealing with public health authorities who monitor such matters, and adjusting their eating habits?

I wanted answers to these questions for the simple reason that, as a journalist, I prefer not to accept government reports at face value. However, in the case of food-borne illness, getting to the "other" side of the story proved much more difficult than might be imagined. For instance, in reporting on the Michigan, California, and Ohio raw milk crackdowns, I was at first unable to obtain the names of the families whose children had supposedly become ill from drinking raw milk. Privacy restrictions prohibited authorities from divulging the names.

So initially I had to take the word of state authorities about what was happening.

As I've mentioned, the owner of California's Organic Pastures, Mark McAfee, told me he had made hospital visits to two of the children supposedly sickened by raw milk. He told me he used his paramedic experience, and some old contacts, to finally track down the two sickest children at Loma Linda Medical Center. But he was loath to provide me with the patient information, and I would have been reluctant myself at that point to try to interview parents who were single-mindedly focused on the health of their children. I knew that, as a parent, the last person I would want to speak with was a journalist trying to write about food-borne illness.

But as time went on, and the children allegedly sickened by raw milk got well, I was able to learn more about the circumstances that led to the major police and legal actions against the producers of raw milk in these three states. The stories I heard were, in important respects, at sharp variance with government versions.

Easter Weekend 2006

As I worked to provide follow-ups about Richard Hebron's case on my blog, several members of the Ann Arbor co-op he was serving contacted me offline. They were mad as hell that the state was trying to deprive them of raw milk—not only because many of them felt it was an essential nutrient in maintaining their health, and in keeping chronic conditions such as colitis and asthma at bay, but because they felt their right to eat foods of their choosing was being violated.

One of these individuals wrote me to say how crazy the whole thing was, especially given the fact that it wasn't even raw milk that had caused the illness triggering the raid. What was this all about? After some back-and-forth, this individual volunteered the identity of the family whose illness had prompted the raid, and how to make contact. So it was that, one morning that November, I was on the phone with Kathryn Corey, a thirty-four-year-old stay-at-home Ann Arbor mom.

She was very upset about the raid on Richard Hebron, and even more upset that events in her household over the previous Easter weekend had set things in motion. Remember, from chapter 1, when I first telephoned Katherine Fedder of the Michigan Department of Agriculture, she told me the sting operation was organized because a family had become ill from raw milk the previous spring? Kathryn Corey said she had thought a lot about what had happened that weekend, had discussed it with her husband, and they had reconstructed the family's meal activity of the weekend and the few days immediately preceding and following the weekend.

Milk was a matter of some consternation and debate in the young Corey household, she told me. She loved raw milk and had, over a period of half a dozen years, become convinced that the presence of "good" bacteria and enzymes, unaffected by the heat of pasteurization, strengthened her immune system and helped in the critical absorption of calcium. She was also certain it reduced the frequency of strep throat and ear infections in her two young children, four-year-old David and seven-year-old Carolyn.

But there has long been a problem if you are a raw milk drinker in Michigan: It is one of the roughly half of states that ban all sales of raw milk—either by retailers or directly by farmers. (I say "roughly half" because the number shifts somewhat based on enforcement of laws and regulations.) In fact, Michigan was the first state in the country to require pasteurization of all milk, in 1947, and thereby make the sale of raw milk illegal. Other states followed in the late 1940s, 1950s, and 1960s.

The good news for Kathryn was that she resided in Ann Arbor, the home of the University of Michigan and long a hotbed not only of liberal politics, but also of alternative health care providers. Cruise around Ann Arbor, a city of 114,000, and you'll see office fronts and billboards offering acupuncture, therapeutic massage, and nutrition counseling.

In 2001, a small group of food-conscious Ann Arbor residents organized something called the Family Farms Cooperative, to help them obtain a regular supply of fresh, locally produced foods that were difficult or impossible to obtain in supermarkets, such as grass-fed beef and eggs from pasture-fed chickens. Within a year, the co-op had 150 family members, and growing demand for an additional product: raw milk. While beef and eggs were no problem to purchase directly from farmers, milk was, because of the explicit state ban.

So the founders of the Family Farms Cooperative took the advice of the Weston A. Price Foundation,[4] an organization founded in memory of a leading nutrition researcher of the 1930s and 1940s who described several healthy traditional populations that consumed large quantities of raw milk. The WAPF advised raw milk advocates in places like Michigan, where sales of raw milk are illegal, to organize herd share or cow share programs. These are legal entities whereby individuals literally buy one or more "shares" in a farmer's dairy herd, usually for something on the order of $50 per. Each share then entitles the holder to a gallon every week or two, in exchange for a "maintenance fee" equivalent to $5 or $10 a gallon to provide food and shelter to the cows. The WAPF even provided the organizers of the Family Farms Cooperative with the paperwork to create their own cow-share arrangement with a farmer 140 miles west of Ann Arbor, Richard Hebron.

Kathryn had heard about the Ann Arbor co-op's cow-share program in 2004, from a friend, and by the time she purchased two shares, the co-op had more than four hundred members. Her two shares entitled her to two gallons of milk every Friday, when Richard Hebron made a delivery to Ann Arbor.

Kathryn began drinking two or three glasses of raw milk a day. She fed it to David and Carolyn. She also made other things from the milk, like kefir and custard.

But as gung-ho as Kathryn was about raw milk, her husband, Joe, was less so. Part of it had to do with the fact that he was a scientist (actually a physics researcher), and, to him, Kathryn's enthusiasm about raw milk wasn't based on proven science. He wasn't a huge milk drinker, but when he did indulge he preferred to stick to the product long since proven by science to be safe— pasteurized and homogenized milk.

On Thursday, April 13, the day before Richard Hebron was due to make his bi-weekly delivery, the Coreys exhausted their raw milk supply at dinner. Knowing that the children usually liked some kind of bedtime snack with milk, "I asked Joe to run out to the Kroger for a half-gallon of milk," Kathryn recalled.

An hour after he returned, "Joe poured some of the pasteurized milk for himself and David for a bedtime snack. Neither Carolyn nor I had any."

About an hour later, "David woke up and complained he had a tummyache. He threw up, but then went back to bed. In the meantime, Joe was up during the night with diarrhea. It was so bad, he didn't go to work the next day."

That next day, Good Friday, Kathryn headed for her raw milk pickup. In the meantime, Joe and David seemed to be on their way to recovery. Kathryn and Joe tried to figure out what might have caused the problem, but nothing stood out, so they figured it was just some kind of "bug" Joe might have picked up from work or David from preschool classes.

Kathryn followed her regular routine that Friday of having a glass of raw milk at mealtimes. She especially enjoyed those first few glasses when the milk was freshest—it had a special creaminess and sweet taste, it seemed. In the meantime, David seemed pretty much himself, and Joe was better, though a bit queasy.

By Easter Sunday, everyone seemed fully mended, recalled Kathryn. "We went out with my parents for a buffet brunch. It was very pleasant."

By the time the Coreys finally returned home, around 5:00 p.m., "We were a bit hungry. So Joe and I did Thai takeout. Not the kids, though," who had some leftovers.

That night was another bad night. Joe's diarrhea was back, worse than ever. And now Carolyn was throwing up, just as David had two nights earlier.

The next day, both father and daughter were still sick. Joe was convinced his diarrhea had been reignited by the Thai food. Carolyn, he thought, had the same bug David had had a few days earlier, since she was vomiting.

Joe decided to call the Washtenaw County Health Department to suggest it check out the Thai restaurant. A health department employee quizzed him about all the foods he and family members had eaten over the previous few days. In addition to the Thai food, he related what they had eaten at the restaurant brunch. Joe also mentioned that David and Carolyn had been sick as well, and that the family drank both pasteurized milk and raw milk.

The health worker called back a few days later to let Joe know that the Thai restaurant hadn't had any other problems with sick customers. Though Carolyn's vomiting stretched out through the following Friday, that seemed to be the end of the matter. The illnesses were over, and there was no further follow-up from public health officials.

At least there was no further follow-up that the Coreys were aware of. But the county public health officials had passed the information about the family's illnesses on to the Michigan Department of Agriculture. Its officials quickly concluded that the Corey children had become ill from raw milk, and put in motion the plan that led to the launch of the sting against Richard Hebron and the Family Farms Co-op.

But in reconstructing the events six months after the fact, Kathryn explained to me, she was now convinced her children and husband had become sick not from raw milk, but from the pasteurized milk Joe had purchased at the grocery store that Thursday evening before Easter. How could she be so sure? Simple, she explained. She was the only family member who hadn't become ill that weekend, and also the only family member who hadn't consumed the pasteurized milk. Everyone else had. Joe, in particular, had had more of the pasteurized milk that Sunday evening when he ate Thai food.

Unfortunately, she hadn't realized the pasteurized milk connection before disposing of the milk carton after the Easter weekend. Add to that evidence the fact that the MDA, which had acquired milk from the Family Farms Cooperative for six months before its sting operation by having an undercover agent pose as a member, never found evidence of pathogens in the milk from Richard Hebron.

Needless to say, when I wrote about the Corey family's experiences on my blog, it created a spate of angry comments.

"So I suppose the Michigan Department of Health will issue an apology, promptly pay damages and issue a press release that absolves the producer from causing the problem?" wrote Paul E. Peldyak. "Not too much to ask, is it?"

"My family has been drinking raw milk for 10 years," stated Carolyn Hejkal. "When I first heard the story of what began the MDA's investigation, I thought it probably would sound about like that when it finally came to light."

Dan Corrigan said, "It's funny, years ago I used to fear drinking raw milk. Now I fear drinking pasteurized milk. When I run out of raw milk, I simply go without drinking milk."[5]

Such cynicism was understandable. The government of Michigan had apparently carried out a major criminal operation against a dairy farmer based on incomplete information and erroneous assumptions.

Labor Day Weekend 2006, Marietta, California

Mary McGonigle-Martin was an unabashed health nut. The forty-eight-year-old high school guidance counselor avoided sugar and white flour and ate lots of vegetables and fruits. She took an assortment of nutritional supplements and occasionally did detoxification "cleanses" whereby she consumed various herbs and reduced her food intake, to help her body rid itself of toxins.

In early August, she was feeling especially good, and credited a just-completed one-month cleanse. She felt so good, in fact, she wanted to do something healthy for her seven-year-old son, Chris. He was a pretty normal kid, but he showed symptoms of attention deficit disorder (ADD), along with sensitivity to certain foods. One of the foods that seemed to especially bother him was milk. "Every morning, he'd wake up congested."

She already had him eating salads and avoiding the sugar and fast food many of his friends consumed. She had also been reading recently on the Internet about raw milk, and how it seemed to help relieve ADD symptoms in children. In her reading, she learned about Organic Pastures Dairy Co., the Fresno, California, dairy that specialized in producing raw milk. She had been impressed by its Web site's description of how it used mobile milking stations to avoid milking the cows in the barn, where conditions could be unsanitary and the milk could become contaminated with pathogens.

California is at the opposite end of the spectrum from Michigan when it comes to unpasteurized milk. It is one of only eight states that allow at least some retailers to sell raw milk (Pennsylvania, Connecticut, Maine, Washington, New Mexico, Arizona, and Utah are the others). Organic Pastures had been aggressively marketing to local health food stores and Whole Foods outlets to carry its milk, butter, and cream—with so much success that, by the summer of 2006, the dairy accounted for nearly 90 percent of California's raw milk sales; more than thirty thousand Californians a day consumed its raw milk.

So one day in early August, Mary stood in front of the dairy refrigerator at the nearby Sprouts Health Food Store in Temecula, debating with herself about whether she should introduce Organic Pastures raw milk into Chris's diet. She thought back to how much she had enjoyed drinking raw milk in the 1980s—until the dairy she purchased it from discontinued raw milk production because the state determined that some of its milk was contaminated with salmonella (although Mary never got sick, nor had anyone she knew).

And that's what had her hesitating—the knowledge that raw milk can become contaminated, that numerous incidents of contamination during the late 1800s and early 1900s had led a number of cities, and then, later in the century, entire states, eventually to require pasteurization. But farmers had so much more knowledge about sanitation now than in those days, she thought. Organic Pastures wouldn't be serving thousands of people every day if there was a serious risk of contamination.

So she reached into the dairy case, pulled out a half-gallon of Organic Pastures raw skim milk, read the warning label that the absence of pasteurization meant it could be harmful to pregnant mothers, the elderly, and young children, and put it in her cart. She began serving it to Chris and drinking it herself. "The results were pretty amazing," she says. "All the symptoms of congestion disappeared."

On Friday, September 1, she was back at Sprouts doing some shopping in anticipation of the upcoming Labor Day weekend. She bought another half-gallon of Organic Pastures raw skim milk, along with some organic red leaf lettuce and organic raw spinach, and checked out.

Over the next two days, Saturday and Sunday, she and Chris indulged in the tasty milk. Her husband, Tony, passed. On Monday, Labor Day, she made a salad for lunch, using the lettuce and spinach she had purchased, and served it to Chris together with the milk.

Late the next afternoon, Tuesday, Chris complained about a headache and feeling nauseous. Mary took his temperature, and it was 101. To keep track of what happened over the ensuing days, Mary and Tony kept a journal. In March 2007, after Mary had by chance come across my blog, she forwarded the journal to me. Once I'd read through it, I asked her if I could publish it on my blog, and she approved the idea. Be forewarned—it is not a pretty picture, and it gets less and less pretty as time goes on. Here is how she recorded the next several days:

> **9/6, Wednesday:** Chris woke in the morning with a fever, ate sparingly, did not attend school. He was lethargic all morning, slept from 12:00 noon until 3:00 p.m. After his nap, he appeared better, ate a normal amount of dinner. At bedtime he had a loose bowel movement and also woke up during the night and again had a loose bowel movement.
>
> **9/7, Thursday:** Chris ate a light breakfast and shortly thereafter began a regimen of loose and watery bowel movements until noon. The pace of the bowel movements increased thereafter, occurring approximately every 15–20 minutes. He also vomited at 10:00 a.m., 12:30 and 3:00 p.m.
>
> The diarrhea became so common that Chris began counting every trip to the bathroom. The 16th bowel movement was primarily slimy mucus—no feces.
>
> The diarrhea and vomiting continued throughout the afternoon and into the evening. At 8:00 p.m., we noticed what appeared to be blood in his stool. We lined the toilet with a plastic bag to capture the next stool—however, this next trip to the toilet netted only blood (approximately 1/8 cup).
>
> At 9:30 p.m. we arrived at the Emergency Room, Kaiser Hospital, Riverside. The vomiting continued; stool, blood, and urine samples were taken; an IV was inserted. Chris was given an anti-vomit medication to help him sleep in the ER.
>
> **9/8, Friday:** Chris was admitted into Kaiser Hospital, Riverside, at approximately 5:00 a.m. Later that morning was the first time we met Dr. A. He arrived with two resident doctors and we heard a very specific explanation regarding his thoughts about presenting symptoms.
>
> He explained to the residents (and to us) that the presenting

symptoms did not allow a determination of bacteria or virus. He stated that the blood and urine samples continued to come back negative. He also informed us that the stool "cultures" would not be available until Monday or Tuesday.

He examined one of Chris's bowel movements and overruled the possibility of salmonella, due to lack of darkness and lack of mucus.

He also stated explicitly to the resident doctors that at no time should Chris be given antibiotics until the cause of the presenting symptoms was identified. He stated that giving antibiotics could make things much worse if this was *E. coli* O157:H7.

Dr. A also stated that morphine could not be administered for my son's cramping because if it was a virus it could cause him to become constipated.

Chris continued to have diarrhea every fifteen to thirty minutes for the entire day and evening. He experienced cramps with each trip to the toilet. During this day, the vomiting, cramping, and diarrhea were manageable.

The absence of a "smoking gun"—an identifiable pathogen in Chris—was something that would persist through the entire traumatic episode. But that didn't stop the medical personnel from coming to their own conclusions. Several times after Mary and Chris arrived at Riverside Hospital, doctors asked her to review what Chris had eaten over the previous few days. She went over the list—raw spinach, red lettuce, zucchinis, carrots . . . and raw milk. . . . When she hit the raw milk, the "uh-huhs" were replaced with a deafening silence. It was as if she could feel backs stiffening and attitudes hardening. Sometimes there were remarks or exasperated questions, in front of Chris, about her carelessness or poor judgment in serving her son raw milk.

At some point—Mary is not sure exactly when—physicians relayed information to local public health authorities about her son having consumed raw milk. The physicians may not have known what made Chris sick, but these authorities were sure they did.

In any event, Chris's condition continued to worsen, as the journal describes.

9/9, Saturday: All presenting symptoms continue throughout the day. Chris vomited before each bowel movement. He was in severe pain.

In the morning, the attending physician wanted us to attempt a food and water challenge. Chris threw up the applesauce and water shortly after consuming it. Shortly thereafter, Chris began experiencing a severe pain on his right side. Doctors suspected appendix. They ruled out appendicitis after two CT scans, but did note an inflammation in his bowel. Dr. B was the attending physician. She consulted with a GI specialist at Riverside and Dr. C at Kaiser, Fontana. She then ordered the first antibiotic: Flagyl. TPN [total parenteral nutrition, or intravenous feeding] was also ordered for nutritional purposes.

During this night, Chris basically sat on the bedside toilet, pillows propped all around him, my wife and I holding him, suffering from the constant urge to defecate. He also developed a rectal prolapse.

9/10, Sunday: In the early morning hours, nurses urged us to request transport to Fontana's pediatric unit, suggesting that a higher level of medical care was necessary for Chris. We heeded their advice. We requested to see the attending physician at approximately 4:00 a.m., and made our request to be transported to Kaiser, Fontana.

We arrived at Kaiser, Fontana at approximately 1:00 p.m. Within a couple of hours of our arrival, a sigmoidoscopy was completed by Dr. C. He diagnosed ulcerative colitis and did a biopsy.

Mary informed Dr. C that Chris had never experienced any bowel issues in his past. Dr. C stated that the colitis had probably been there dormant, but that it *"was odd that the symptoms did come on so quickly."*

A *second* antibiotic was ordered: Claforan.

Within hours of arriving at Kaiser, Fontana, Chris now had the following items flowing through his intravenous feeding tube: TPN, saline solution, and two antibiotics: Flagyl and Claforan.

Note: Up until our fateful trip to Kaiser, Fontana, all blood tests were negative. In fact, his blood work was normal. This is key to understanding how the lack of continuity between doctors in the Kaiser system created this medical disaster for my child. *Within hours of hanging the antibiotics, everything changes.*

9/11, Monday: At 6:00 a.m., blood has been detected in Chris's urine. A final bowel movement is released at 10:30 a.m., which amounts to a mammoth flow of gold liquid gushing out of his rectum, overflowing his diaper and filling a 3x3 absorption pad on the bed.

The attending physician, Dr. D, came into the room shortly after this final bowel movement . . . Dr. D told us that we had a very sick child. She told us that he may have to be moved to the pediatric intensive care unit at Kaiser Sunset and that his illness may involve kidney dialysis. She told us that she is waiting for the next round of blood tests to confirm her suspicion. She ordered a catheter be inserted into his penis for the collection of urine.

Dr. D returned within the hour. She officially diagnosed Chris with HUS (hemolytic uremic syndrome). She informed us that we would immediately be flown to Los Angeles, CA, Kaiser Sunset, where Chris would be admitted to Pediatric Intensive Care.

Note: Dr. A had officially warned of antibiotic treatment and the dangers it posed. He had written his warning into the record. And now, within *hours* of other doctors not heeding his warning, Chris was in medical crisis.

Chris's descent from normal blood labs to HUS diagnosis occurred within *hours* of the second antibiotic being administered. An article published in the *New England Journal of Medicine* in 2000 warns about the dangers of HUS following antibiotic treatment.[6]

Mary and Chris arrived at Kaiser Sunset at approximately 1:30 p.m.

Tony arrived by car shortly thereafter. The attending physicians informed us about the possibility of kidney dialysis. They suggested that some children do not require dialysis, that if Chris continued peeing and his urine turned yellow, it would be a positive sign.

A central line was placed in our son's right shoulder. This would be used for blood draws and the administration of meds and nutrition. . . .

9/12, Tuesday: On this day we met with Dr. P. . . . She talked about HUS and also discussed the medical requirements for Chris to receive dialysis. They included a BUN of over 100, creatinine over 5.0, and renal failure. We were also told that Kaiser Sunset does not do kidney dialysis; that if our son's condition does reach these benchmarks, he would then have to be moved and admitted to Children's Hospital, Los Angeles.

We spent the remainder of this day watching our son's urine output slowly dissipate, while his energy level followed close behind . . .

9/13, Wednesday: Dr. P greeted us with a diagnosis of shigella. She stated that the lab had not isolated the bacteria, however they had found shiga toxin. She explained that shiga toxin is the by-product of *Shigella* dying off. Of course, the antibiotics killed the *Shigella*, if it was *Shigella*, in our son's body, resulting in the toxins being released in his body, which is why antibiotics should not be administered . . . Dr. P also explained, compassionately, that our son's condition would get much worse before it got better. She stated that these shiga-toxins would now march through our son's body for the next ten days. Only then would we be able to assess the long-term damage.

We spent the day monitoring urine output. It was clear that our son's kidneys were shutting down. Every benchmark was being rapidly approached. Tony questioned Dr. P on this day, asking her why we had to wait until our son was drowning in toxins before we could help him with dialysis. Her response was dry and bureaucratic: "Kidney dialysis is a serious intervention with new risks attached to it."

We had spent the last two days watching our son being loaded with fluid and (drugs). Chest X-rays were ordered, and Dr. K informed us that fluid was now gathering on his lungs. Again we wondered about dialysis. Why were we waiting to meet these absurd benchmarks? Dialysis could draw off these excess fluids, as well as lower his BUN and creatinine.

We spent the night watching our worst nightmare unfold. Each hour we measured his urine in the container next to his bed. Each hour it lessened. By morning, nothing. No urine output. Kidney failure.

9/14: At 8:00 a.m., Chris had officially met the benchmarks: BUN—102, creatinine—4.9, kidney failure, and his hemoglobin was 7.1—he would need a blood transfusion. We were told that arrangements were being made for his transfer to Children's Hospital.

We waited for hour after hour. We kept questioning the doctors.

What's the hold-up? It's been five hours. Our son needs dialysis. He needed it two days ago. No one had an answer. No one seemed to care.

Finally, at 1:30 p.m., word came. But it was not what we expected. We were informed that Children's Hospital did not have a bed for our son. . . . There would be a delay. Dr. K told us that they were going to contact UCLA Medical Center to see if there was a bed available.

Tony realized that he could no longer watch this slow-motion, bureaucratic nightmare called "Kaiser Critical Care" attempt to function. He insisted that our son be sent to Loma Linda University Children's Hospital. . . . He eventually convinced the doctors and Kaiser administration to approve the transfer, which happened by the end of that day.

Chris was transferred to Loma Linda Medical Center by helicopter. By the time he reached the hospital, a race began to save the young boy's life. The journal continues:

His breathing was labored. X-rays were taken immediately. Dr. G showed us the pictures and told us that the reason he was breathing so hard was because he had lots of fluid behind his lungs. Pleural effusion. He told us that he would have to place a drainage tube into each side of our son's chest. He explained the risks. We approved the procedure. 1100 cc's drained out of our son over the next few hours, over 5000 cc's over the next three weeks.

Our son also received emergency dialysis that night . . .

9/15, Friday: Our first full day at Loma Linda. Chris received the much-needed blood transfusion. He received dialysis again. He suffered from bad cramps and dry heaves for hours. He was absolutely miserable. After all, this was his eighth day in the hospital. He was absolutely exhausted.

As the day progressed, he got progressively worse. By evening, his chest was pounding. Harder and faster. Harder and faster. 130 beats per minute, 140, 150, 170, 180. At this point, Dr. T came to us and told us that Chris was now in danger of congestive heart failure—a heart attack. She informed us that modern medicine would now have to take over some of Chris's bodily functions—he would have to be intubated to slow down his heart and let him sleep.

We were devastated. It seemed Chris was slipping further and further away.

9/16, Saturday: It was now 2:00 a.m. The ventilator was managing Chris's every breath. He was sedated. On this day he also received plasma, another blood transfusion, kidney dialysis. And much needed rest.

9/20: Chris would spend nearly five full days on the ventilator. His testicles grew to the size of a large grapefruit, his face and extremities were now puffed and abnormal. We stared at our son's face, hour after hour, so swollen that we wouldn't have recognized him on the street had he passed by in that condition . . .

But the boy's condition did improve, though with setbacks along the way.

From this point forward, days turned into weeks. Chris was taken off the ventilator after five days. He could not speak from a swollen throat, more drugs were administered to reduce the swelling. He had to wear a tightly fitted mask (Bi-Pap) over his mouth and nose, forcing oxygen deep into his lungs, due to a partially collapsed lung . . .

9/29: Chris had a seizure due to high blood pressure. He was again intubated. Cat Scan, EEG, MRI, more sedation would follow.

10/1: He was taken off the ventilator at 11:45 p.m. Still suffering from abnormally high blood pressure. Taking medications to stabilize.

Over the next month, Chris gradually improved, and finally, on November 2, he left the hospital to go home. One other thing is important to note about the Martins' experience at Loma Linda. There they met the parents of ten-year-old Lauren Herzog, who had developed symptoms similar to Chris's at about the same time. She had also consumed raw milk. While she didn't experience as much suffering in advance of getting to Loma Linda, she did require kidney dialysis as well. Unlike Chris, she was diagnosed with *E. coli* O157:H7. She was the second child Mark McAfee visited when he came to the hospital on September 25. She also recovered enough during October to be able to go home. More about the cases of Chris Martin and Lauren Herzog later.

The same strain of *E. coli* O157:H7 found in Lauren would be found in four other children who became ill around the same time. All those children only became mildly ill and recovered at home after a few days. Because none of the *E. coli* O157:H7 could be matched to anything found in Mark McAfee's cows, he was allowed to resume operations.

Dayton, Ohio, Spring 2006

In the process of investigating the crackdown on raw milk in Ohio, I met up with Gary Cox, a lawyer with a private law firm in Dayton, who specialized in agriculture cases. He had represented Carol Schmitmeyer (mentioned in chapter 1) before the Ohio Department of Agriculture in her hearing in September 2006, and would represent her afterward in her court appeal of the ODA's decision to revoke her dairy license.

When public health authorities and the ODA were investigating the illnesses in early 2006, she had asked her shareholders to write to the ODA and express support for her and the raw milk she was producing.

Cox sent me about a dozen of those affidavits of support and, lo and behold, two were from individuals who had supposedly become sick from raw milk—cases that the ODA claimed triggered its crackdown on Carol Schmitmeyer and other raw dairy producers. One letter was from Jacob and Carolyn Hall, and read:

> Our son Peter (age four) did have diarrhea, which our pediatrician confirmed as a campylobacter infection. However, I do not believe it is conclusive that it was caused from the raw milk that he consumed. First of all, every member of our family drank the milk, including our one-year-old daughter and six-year-old son. Peter was the only person who was ill during this time.
>
> In addition, our pediatrician, as well as the woman who contacted me from the Public Health Service, informed us that campylobacter is often contracted through feces from animals, especially birds. We live in a neighborhood with a large number of mature trees and as a consequence, a large population of birds, even in the winter months.
>
> Our son Peter had eaten a handful of snow from a shrub in our front yard on the way to the car two days before he became ill with diarrhea. We believe that this could easily have caused the diarrhea.

It was about 50 degrees outside, there were plenty of birds and squirrels around, and the snow was melting. There could have been droppings anywhere in the yard from these animals.

Nobody else in our family ate any snow, but the other members all drank the milk. Peter was the only person who became ill. This information alone is enough for us to doubt the association of raw milk and his illness.

We urge you to consider the complete story behind this illness and not make a conclusion based on vague, incomplete information. We feel that our family was used to further your agenda against raw milk. Instead of helping us, as we believe government agencies should, you used our situation to further your cause by placing our family's information in the newspaper without our knowledge. In addition, the information included in the newspaper was incomplete.

One of the articles this parent was apparently referring to stated, "Agriculture officials began investigating the Schmitmeyer farm after a 63-year-old man and a 4-year-old boy who drank raw milk from the farm became ill with campylobacter infections in January."[7]

The sixty-three-year-old man, Floyd R. Hilt of Springfield, Ohio, also wrote in, noting, "It was stated in the newspaper that I was in good health prior to contracting the bacteria. . . . [But] I had a compromised immune system before I contracted the bacteria."

His letter detailed his various ailments—edema in the ankles and legs, shortness of breath, as well as being on a number of prescription drugs. After becoming ill in January 2006 and being admitted to a hospital, he was diagnosed as having an infection from campylobacter.

I questioned the raw milk being the cause, as my wife was drinking it also, along with other family members, with no problems at all. I personally questioned if I could have picked up this bacteria at work. I work at a Drug and Alcohol Rehab Center. My wife questioned a bologna sandwich she had caught me eating, thinking it had been in the refrigerator for some time. We questioned whether it was a burger from Wendy's, or from chicken we had eaten. The Health Department even said they had seen an increase in the bacteria in raw vegetables. We began to question everything we had eaten or drank.

Mr. Hilt may have been questioning things closely, but he seemed to be asking more questions than the public health officials. They very quickly assumed the culprit was raw milk—a conclusion that all too often seems to be made automatically, before any investigation has begun or any scientific evidence has been analyzed.

CHAPTER THREE

Why Are We Still Debating Pasteurization?

Give me a break with all of this raw milk hoohah. Milk from a cow or a human breast is sterile, unless the cow or human has mastitis. The "beneficial microbes" in cow's milk that some claim to be so beneficial are skin contaminants from the cow's teat. Have you ever known a child that died from an infection caused by contaminated food, milk, or water? I have. Why take a chance on raw milk when in several studies by universities, raw milk has never been scientifically proven to be better for you than pasteurized milk, in fact exactly the opposite has been found. Or do you believe in the scientific process at all? Louis Pasteur would be shocked.

From "A Nurse in NY," posted on my blog[1]

Most of the people who post comments on my blog consume raw milk, and say their health has improved as a result. But there's a significant minority, like "A Nurse in NY," who are afraid of raw milk, and can't understand, in any event, why people would even consider taking an action counter to the work of Louis Pasteur.

I have little doubt that "A Nurse in NY" really is a nurse. Her view is common in the medical establishment. Aside from questions about its technical accuracy—over milk's state when it comes out of the cow—her overall attitude, essentially that "food is food," pervades our society.

But the fact that this view is increasingly being called into question—evidenced not only by the exploding growth in raw milk consumption, but by the growing popularity of the local food, organic food, and so-called Slow Food movements—may help explain why the government is waging a war on raw milk at this particular moment in time, in the early twenty-first century, more than a century after Louis Pasteur devised his process[2] and fifty or more years after pasteurization had become almost universally accepted by our society. (Today we also have ultra-high-temperature pasteurization, which involves heating the milk to 250 degrees Fahrenheit or more for up to a couple seconds, and has the effect of essentially sterilizing it, and thus extending its shelf life by many weeks.)

It's been impossible to obtain a true explanation for the sudden assault on raw milk, since the state and federal agencies involved in the raids and enforcement actions in Ohio, Michigan, and California wouldn't even acknowledge that their suddenly high-profile actions constituted a change in approach. And they refused to participate in public debates or discussions about the subject. For example, when a Washington radio talk show host invited the FDA to send a representative to discuss raw milk with several proponents of raw milk in August 2007, the agency refused the invitation, according to the host, saying, "This is not a debatable issue."[3]

Almost two years later, in February 2009, a contingent of a dozen FDA officials, led by Division of Plant and Dairy Food Safety head John Sheehan, pulled out of a special symposium on the alleged dangers of raw milk ("Raw Milk Consumption: An Emerging Public Health Threat?") sponsored by the main industry trade association concerned with food-borne illness, the International Association for Food Protection. IAFP officials told me that the FDA attendees canceled the Friday before the Tuesday event, without explanation; The only plausible reason I could come up with was that they were scared off by learning I was going to be there, along with four representatives of the Weston A. Price Foundation, including its president, Sally Fallon Morell. (An FDA spokesperson subsequently said Sheehan was concerned because "FDA is presently involved in litigation with a raw milk vendor, and while that matter is pending, it was considered advisable to not discuss matters which might relate to the litigation." He refused to say which litigation Sheehan was referring to or when it may have started. Presumably the litigation was going on when Sheehan agreed to be a speaker at the conference, and have his name included in the program.)

However, by assessing what key federal officials were saying publicly about alleged raw milk illnesses, especially about the California illnesses attributed to Organic Pastures Dairy Co., it is possible to gain insight into the agency's official positions. In doing that, I learned that the government's arguments in the early 2000s were not entirely different from a debate that percolated during the late 1800s, after Louis Pasteur came up with his pathogen-killing heat treatment process for wine—namely, is it germs that make us sick, or does our immune system's inability to fend off certain germs at certain times lead to illness?

By early 2007, the California children's illnesses, which included the two most serious cases of all those supposedly caused by raw milk, were attracting an increasing amount of attention—from government regulators, the children's parents, and ordinary citizens. In testimony to Maryland legislators opposing proposed legislation that would have lifted the state's prohibition on all sales of raw milk, and allowed farmers to sell directly to consumers, the FDA's top expert on dairy products, John Sheehan, used the California illnesses as evidence to support his position:

> An outbreak of food-borne illness involving *E. coli* O157:H7 . . . occurred in California last year. This outbreak was determined by California to likely be caused by a dairy owned by a raw milk advocate. The evidence linking these illnesses to this dairy was strong enough to prompt California authorities to order the milk to be recalled. According to California authorities, all three victims in this outbreak were children and all three were hospitalized.

(Actually, Sheehan's statement was at odds with what California officials reported—that six children were thought to have been sickened, and two were hospitalized.)

Maybe because the evidence against raw milk in the Michigan and Ohio cases was so questionable, Sheehan didn't mention them, and they didn't come up in FDA presentations about the dangers of raw milk. However, the tough tactics used against Gary Oaks rated a brief mention in an FDA presentation. In a January PowerPoint presentation on its Web site, "Raw-Milk Associated Public Health Risks,"[4] the agency dedicated a slide to Oaks's Double O Farm, saying it was "distributing milk to shareholders of farm's cows at various drop-off points in [the] Cincinnati area. . . . The Ohio Department of Agriculture, Kentucky Public Health Department, and USFDA confiscated milk from truck and shareholders' bottles in a Cincinnati parking lot on March 6, 2006."

In his Maryland testimony, Sheehan explained his opposition to raw milk in terms that regulators most often rely on—fear and protection.

> Raw milk is inherently dangerous and should not be consumed. Raw milk continues to be a source of food-borne illness and even a

cause of death within the United States. . . . FDA encourages everyone charged with protecting the public health to prevent the sale of
raw milk to consumers . . .

His biggest concern, he said, was for children.

When one reads all the literature available on the association
between *E. coli* O157:H7, HUS [hemolytic uremic syndrome], and
raw milk, one wonders whether children themselves would choose
to drink raw milk if they knew that raw milk might make them
very ill, cause them to lose their kidneys, or even kill them. Given a
child's enthusiasm for life, I doubt very much that they would. Since
children cannot and do not know about such matters, however, it
is incumbent upon those of us who do know and are responsible
for protecting them to ensure that the likelihood of their contracting food-borne disease from any food, including the milk that they
drink, is an ever-diminishing prospect.

In raising the specter of sick children, Sheehan was coming full circle, back
to the original reason for implementing pasteurization on an ever-wider
basis—to protect those least able to protect themselves.

But that still didn't answer the question of why now. He may inadvertently have alluded to the reason when he made this concluding statement:

Despite the claims of raw milk advocates, raw milk is not a magi-
cal elixir possessing miraculous curative properties. Pasteurization
destroys pathogens and most other vegetative microbes which
might be expected and have been shown to be present in milk.
Pasteurization does not appreciably alter the nutritive value of milk.
Claims to the contrary by raw milk advocates are without scientific
support.

What he was suggesting, without admitting something that would
no doubt have been very painful to him, was that increasing numbers of
consumers were listening to "the claims of raw milk advocates," and in the
process ignoring the arguments of government officials like Sheehan—
about both the dangers of raw milk and the nutritional value of the pasteurized kind—and seeking out the unpasteurized version.

On my blog,[5] the reaction to the posting of Mary McGonigle-Martin's journal (quoted at length in the previous chapter) provided ample evidence of cynicism about the FDA's position. Certainly many readers were very sympathetic to her, at least initially. Chris Martin seemed at first glance like a poster boy for pasteurization.

"Mary and Tony, Oh my God, your story has left me shaking. I hope you consider writing a book about this," wrote Elizabeth McInerney, in a typical response.

But once the shock over the details of her ordeal wore off, readers had questions and concerns. Some expressed skepticism about whether it was actually raw milk that had made Chris sick.

"I'm very sorry that such a young child had to go through this," wrote Kirsten. "The thing is, you can't be sure that the raw milk caused this. The onset of symptoms is the average three to four days, but onset can occur in as little as one day. . . . There is a small chance that something besides food could have caused this awful condition. I understand the inclination to associate it with the milk, but there isn't any hard laboratory evidence to back this up."

Ken Conrad said he was especially upset. "Mary and Tony Martin's story of their son was truly a gut-wrenching one for me to read," he said. The reason, he explained, was that his wife had gone through a horrible childbirth twenty years earlier, made worse by inappropriate drugs. In the end, she died, while her twins survived. Ken brought the two babies home to join their two older children.

> Once at home and being an organic dairy farmer I fed the babies whole raw Jersey milk mixed with raw honey and diluted with fresh spring water. Angela and Jacob will be 20 years of age on October 3 of this year; they have not been vaccinated, have not seen a doctor since their birth, and have not received prescription or over-the-counter medications of any kind.
>
> The two eldest children on the other hand, as a result of a desire to follow the doctor's orders, were fed formula and vaccinated. They experienced recurrent ear and gastrointestinal infections accompanied by severe diarrhea. They received antibiotics as well as numerous over-the-counter medications, have had tubes in their ears and were hospitalized due to the above infections.

His conclusion: "If someone were to ask me today if raw milk were a cause of disease, I would have to unequivocally say no."

Beyond that, a number of readers with knowledge about health and illness questioned a fundamental premise of our medical and public health establishments: that germs inevitably cause disease. According to these readers' argument, people certainly can and do get sick from pathogens, but they do so because of failures in their own immune systems, rather than because the germs are so strong.

Laurie[6] described an ordeal she went through with physicians when her young daughter became ill after receiving an MMR (measles, mumps, rubella) vaccination, and then nearly died after being given antibiotics to counter her illness. "I subsequently learned a great deal about vaccinations," she wrote, "and about the immune system—and about the cause/s of what we call 'disease,' which took me very far from the simplistic and hyper-mechanical 'good-guy drug vs. bad-guy microbe' thinking, which is the premise of the allopathic medical model."

She added that she remains a fan of milk produced by Organic Pastures Dairy Co. in California:

> My continuing good opinion of OP milk is based on years of looking ever more deeply into the factors which create or undermine health. One of the first things I learned was that the whole "germ theory," as it is simplistically taught to us, is flawed—based as it is on Pasteur's conclusions, which were a bastardization of the work of French biologist Antoine Bechamp, whose far more comprehensive conclusions yielded the premise that "pathogens" are actually secondary to the "terrain"—in a sense, bacteria are actually a life form that come into being due to the conditions in which they are found—from an even-more-mysterious life element which Bechamp called a "microzyma." It seems that under different conditions within a petri dish, an organism recognized as the "bacillus considered to be causative for a particular disease" can mutate into an entirely different type of bacteria or microbiological unit considered causative for something different. [This] was of interest to me because, while I still understand that our systems are not designed to prevail against a sudden onslaught/intake of unfamiliar pathogenic bacterial life forms, that bacteria [are] not automatically

the causative agents of illness and so "anti" biotics and "germ"icidal agents are not the cure-all panacea they are promoted as. This is a complicated subject—however, I believe that eliminating the fungus (which antibiotics install in us) and restoring the presence of beneficial "bacteria" throughout the intestines and body is very key to health. I use a variety of foods and supplements to work toward establishing that condition. Certainly OP (Organic Pastures) milk is a highly valued part of that process in the lives of my children and family—however it can be achieved by other means if someone believes that beneficial bacteria is part of the intrinsic picture of best possible health.

All of this debate and discussion about the origin of disease prompted me to do additional reading and research as well.

Like nearly every other kid growing up in late-twentieth-century America, I had learned the stories of such accomplished scientists and inventors as Louis Pasteur, Eli Whitney, and Alexander Graham Bell—of how their dramatic breakthroughs made possible the Industrial Revolution and, ultimately, the wonderfully safe and convenient life I was able to enjoy. Of all the stories about such innovators, the one about how Louis Pasteur developed a heating process used to rid milk of bad germs always seemed most dramatic. In the context of the epidemics that killed many thousands of children in America's big cities, Louis Pasteur's technique of heating a substance like milk to get rid of bad germs and significantly reduce the incidence of such dangerous diseases as tuberculosis and diphtheria must have seemed like magic. It's easy to see why, based on that single development, he became something of a scientific folk hero.

As I read more about the problems of milk in the nineteenth century, though, I came to understand that the tale wasn't at all so simple. One of the best books to set the context is *The Untold Story of Milk*,[7] by Connecticut naturopath Ron Schmid. He makes the point that raw milk—whether from cows, goats, sheep, or camels—was consumed for centuries with little or no problem.

It was when America was being transformed by the Industrial Revolution of the early and mid-1800s that the problems began. As masses of people migrated from countryside to the city in search of high-paying jobs, there were businesspeople who brought cows in from the country as well to provide basic foods—alcohol for adults and milk for children—ironically, from the same source. First, corn and barley would be fermented to make vodka and whiskey, and the leftover grains, their nutrients depleted, would be fed to cows housed in adjoining buildings.

These were the first feedlots, the first major effort at agricultural industrialization based on exploiting farm animals on a large scale, for purely economic reasons, to maximize profits. Here is how Robert Hartley, an advocate for the poor who investigated the urban dairy industry, described the situation in the early 1840s, for anyone who is "still skeptical as to the pernicious quality of the milk":

> If the wind is in the right quarter, he will smell the dairy a mile off; and on reaching it, his visual and nasal organs will, without any affectation of squeamishness, be so offended at the filth and effluvia which abounds, that still-slop milk will probably become the object of his unutterable loathing the remainder of his life. His attention will probably be first drawn to a huge distillery, sending out its tartarian fumes, and, blackened with age and smoke, casting a somber air all around. Contiguous thereto, he will see numerous low, flat pens, in which many hundreds of cows, owned by different persons, are closely huddled together, amid confined air, and the stench of their own excrements. He will also see the various appendages and troughs to conduct and receive the hot slush from the still with which to gorge the stomachs of these unfortunate animals, and all within an area of a few hundred yards.[8]

Hartley described further how the cows at first didn't care for the distillery slop. The dairy owners would then deprive them of water, so the cows ate the slop to satisfy their thirst. For a few months, their milk production soared, but eventually they became diseased—their teeth falling out—and unable to stand. At that point, they were sold for slaughter, and their meat sold as beef.

Because there was so little understanding about the connection between sanitation and communicable disease, few objected to the ongoing abuse. But even without scientific evidence, people like Hartley felt certain that the connection was there.

> Let the parent who feeds his children with milk from the dairies at Brooklyn, visit those places and look for once into the buildings where the cows are crowded together with scarcely space enough

between them to allow a milkman to pass; let him take two long breaths of that filthy atmosphere, from which the poor animals are not permitted to stir for weeks and months; let him smell of the heart-sickening rum-broth upon which these abused creatures are compelled almost exclusively to feed—each drinking from fifteen to thirty gallons a day; let him examine the stumps of the teeth corroded down to the gums by the acrid fluids generated from the unwholesome food; let him learn that some of these animals, becoming in a single season unfit for the dairy, are fattened partly upon the same poisonous composition, and killed and carried into market to be eaten by himself and family; and then let him say whether he will patronize such nefarious establishments.

Nothing can be more certain, than that the quality of the milk is greatly influenced by the state of the health of the animal producing it; and where such immense quantities of a mischievous material as fifteen or thirty gallons are made to pass through the organs of a single animal in twenty-four hours, it is impossible that the functions of the organs should be performed in a perfect manner. The milk thus produced might almost as well be taken directly from the distillery, without the ceremony of straining it through the blood-vessels of a sickly cow.[9]

He followed up these descriptions with examples of individuals becoming ill from drinking the distillery milk—individuals who had previously drunk carefully produced milk from rural farms, without problems.

Enter Louis Pasteur, the father of microbiology and the originator of the health principle that has guided much of medicine since the 1860s—the so-called germ theory. This is the idea that microscopic bacteria are responsible for making us sick.

All of which got me wanting to learn more about Louis Pasteur. The more I read, the more I came to realize a number of things about him that I hadn't fully understood.

First, milk was a minor part of his scientific exploits. When I examined biographies of Pasteur, I found that milk received barely a mention. In the 551-page tome *Louis Pasteur,* pasteurization of milk received mention on only one page, after a long discussion about how the process actually originated with the scientist's efforts during the 1860s to find a way to help the

French wine industry deal with problems of wine spoilage during transport. He identified various bacteria that were part of the spoilage and came up with the technique of heating the wine for a few moments without air to between 140 and 212 degrees Fahrenheit.

Despite elaborate demonstrations to show that the pasteurized wine tasted better after shipping than nonpasteurized wine, there were acrimonious debates in France about whether the heating altered the taste of the wine. A blue-ribbon panel finally sided with Pasteur that the wine's taste wasn't adversely affected. Ironically, France's wine industry grew disillusioned with pasteurization within a few decades.

> The experiments with heating wine succeeded because heating does kill microbes. Yet, applied to wine, pasteurization had neither the success nor the scope Pasteur anticipated. By the end of the century, phylloxera (insects that destroy grape vines) was to do more harm to French wine and wine trade than the diseases of cloudiness and bitterness that Pasteur had been able to control. The practice of heating fell into disuse among the vintners, who experienced far greater distress.... [But] the heating process was soon to be applied to other foodstuffs, as well as to other beverages, first and foremost to milk and beer.[10]

Actually, Pasteur's most notable accomplishment likely came nearly twenty years after his wine pasteurization project. He moved on from pasteurization to vaccination. Probably his most famous experiment occurred in 1881, when he inoculated twenty-four sheep, one goat, and six cows against anthrax in farm animals, and then injected live virus into both the "protected" animals and a control group of the same number of animals. The experiment went just as intended—the protected animals were fine and the control group's animals were dead or dying.[11]

Pasteur's experiment helped kick off what became known as the Golden Age of Bacteriology from 1880 to 1900, during which time more than a dozen important pathogens were identified, including malaria, tuberculosis, cholera, diphtheria, and tetanus.[12]

Despite all the excitement about these discoveries, there was, in fact, dissension from Pasteur's germ theory from some of the most prominent scientists of the day, nearly all of whom were French. Antoine Béchamp argued for the cell theory, in an attempt to explain the obvious—that pathogens didn't make everyone sick. In his view, some people's cellular systems were specially equipped to handle these pathogens without becoming ill.

A similarly fundamental rift occurred with the French physiologist Claude Bernard. He preached about the *milieu interieur,* described by Ron Schmid in *The Untold Story of Milk* as "the internal environment the individual brings to the battleground of infectious disease—that which creates resistance, inner strength and, for some, complete immunity. The great debate in science and medicine during the latter half of the nineteenth century was about microbes versus milieu in the etiology of infectious disease. At center stage stood Bernard and Louis Pasteur."[13]

A biography of Pasteur even describes a Bernard physiology course that Pasteur audited: "Pasteur did not pay sufficient attention to one of the most important concepts put forward by Claude Bernard, that of the internal environment. The notes he had taken on this subject when he audited the physiologist's course did not trigger anything in his imagination; and so he did not push his studies in this area any further, although this might have led him to discover the antibodies or the immune system in general." [14]

As Lebre summarizes, "On Pasteur's side is an exogenous concept, in which the microbe invades the body. On Bernard's side, disease is due to a disturbance of the internal environment."[15]

Perhaps the most significant voice of dissension, though, came from a Russian immunologist, Elie Metchnikoff. During the 1880s, he came up with a radical theory: that certain white blood cells could engulf and destroy harmful bodies such as bacteria. Most of the leading scientists of the West, including Pasteur, scorned Metchnikoff and his, to them, improbable theory.[16]

Metchnikoff and Pasteur eventually patched things up, to the extent that Pasteur gave him an appointment at the Pasteur Institute, where he remained for the rest of his life. But lending support to his seemingly radical theory about immunity was the Nobel Prize Metchnikoff won in 1908.

As a new century unfolded, though, Pasteur's viewpoint became ever more dominant, and those of Bernard and Metchnikoff ever less influential. The unhappy rivalry can be seen in the unfolding history of milk during the twentieth century.

Because of the faith people had in the nutritional power of raw milk, the notion of heat-treating it was slow to catch on. But by the early 1900s, as disease outbreaks continued to ravage large cities, pasteurization was increasingly introduced into them. The first city to begin requiring it was

Chicago, followed by New York, Boston, Philadelphia, Milwaukee, and San Francisco. Yet public acceptance came more slowly, in significant measure because much of the conventional medical wisdom of the day claimed benefits for unpasteurized milk. In Chicago, for example, "It took eight years of political contestation for Chicago to mandate full pasteurization in 1916," recounts one local history.[17]

The forerunner of the Mayo Clinic placed great emphasis on raw milk as an antidote to many illnesses. Here is how a physician described his approach in an article in a 1929 dairy magazine:

> For fifteen years the writer has employed the certified [raw] milk treatment in various diseases and during the past ten he had a small sanitarium devoted principally to this treatment. The results obtained in various types of disease have been so uniformly excellent that one's conception of disease and its alleviation is necessarily changed.[18]

A very different perspective appears in a report from the Centers for Disease Control, one that interprets the advent of pasteurization as a slow but inevitable reaction to disease outbreaks:

> Pasteurization of milk . . . was also adopted slowly over many years. At the turn of the last century, cows' milk was recognized as the source of a large number of different infections, including typhoid fever, bovine tuberculosis, diphtheria, and severe streptococcal infections. A commercial pasteurizer was patented in Germany in 1893, and, by 1900, a standard set of pasteurization conditions were defined, based on the time and temperature required to inactivate *Mycobacterium tuberculosis,* which was thought to be the most heat-resistant pathogen. However, pasteurization was opposed because it was believed that it might be used to market dirtier milk and also because of fears that it might affect the nutritional value of milk; therefore, the technology was implemented slowly. For some, the best way to prevent infections spread through milk was to pay scrupulous attention to the health of animals and to create sanitary conditions for the milk production process. This "certification movement" led to substantial improvements in dairy conditions. However, recurrent outbreaks of illness traced to some certified

dairies clearly indicated a need for pasteurization. Initially, different jurisdictions adopted either improved sanitation or pasteurization. The requirements of the Public Health Service Standard Milk Ordinance in 1927 combined the two strategies: first, milk was to be graded based on a variety of sanitation measures; second, only Grade A milk could be pasteurized. By the end of the 1940s pasteurization was heavily promoted throughout the industry and became the norm. Now, 99% of fresh milk consumed in the United States is pasteurized, Grade A.[19]

When the report says that "pasteurization was heavily promoted throughout the industry," it means milk processors exploited the growing official movement toward pasteurization to promote the establishment of processing plants. The emerging industry pushed not only pasteurization but also homogenization as a means to prevent cream from floating to the top of the milk. Not until the late 1940s, however, did Michigan become the first state to require pasteurization of all milk, and in effect outlaw raw milk—based on a huge marketing push by processors to overcome resistance, first to pasteurization and then to homogenization.

The different interpretations of how we become ill, and how pasteurization developed, underscore the reality that we don't fully understand infectious disease. In other words, much of what we are told about illness is based as much on theory as on a full understanding of the process. So in reviewing the history, I came to understand that Pasteur was responsible for developing not only a theory to explain the world of health and disease that permeates our modern-day view of how and why people become ill, but a very special theory. His was a theory people could easily understand and relate to. A theory in which there was an easily identifiable villain: the germs.

Pasteur's argument that germs invade the body and cause disease is visible in nearly every aspect of our daily lives—in the advertisements of mouthwashes that promise to kill all bacteria, in the everyday explanation of colds and fevers from doctors and friends alike that "You caught a bug," to the requirement that foods such as almonds and apple cider be pasteurized, to the ongoing campaign that our food be "zapped" by low doses of radiation to eliminate pathogens.

Probably the biggest boosts came from the simple fact that people could see dramatic evidence that Pasteur's theory "worked." Schmid notes that,

"With widespread pasteurization, [the infant mortality rate] fell . . . from a rate of 160 deaths under one year of age for every 1,000 births in 1906 to 90 in 1916." Some advocates of raw milk don't like to acknowledge pasteurization's role, but Schmid observes, "Advocates for raw milk should understand, however, that sloppily produced and contaminated raw milk in America's circa 1900 cities caused considerable disease and death. Pasteurization began as an apparent solution to this acute problem."[20]

The "miracle" of pasteurization was followed up by vaccination in the early 1900s, and the development of antibiotics in the 1930s, which "cured" all kinds of previously dangerous illnesses, from tonsilitis to bronchitis to pneumonia, not to mention life-threatening infections from serious cuts and wounds. During World War II, the seemingly miraculous effects of penicillin and sulfa drugs were experienced by soldiers, who spoke excitedly to their relatives back home.

Because the germ theory is so widely accepted today, it is difficult to appreciate that during Pasteur's early professional life, in the 1840s and 1850s, it was a completely radical idea. No one knew exactly how disease originated, and because of the void that existed, there were all kinds of theories. Some had diseases appearing spontaneously. A variation on this theme had them appearing as acts of God. Another theory was that disease sprang from corpses, somehow transmitted through the air to living people.

Pasteur personally experienced the trials and tragedy associated with diseases common during that era—two of his five children died of typhoid. But as Pasteur's exploits were publicized, his germ theory gained more and more credence. First, there was his success with heating wine to retard fermentation, which for a time helped the huge French wine industry reduce spoilage. This concept was extended by food producers to milk and beer and, during the twentieth and early twenty-first centuries, to apple cider and other juices and, eventually, to almonds. Then there was his five years of work to track down disease in silkworms, which saved the French silk industry. And then his experiments with vaccines, most notably in heading off rabies and anthrax.

I was clued in to the continuing debate over the germ theory by several commenters on my blog. One of them, Miguel, a dairy farmer with a deep understanding of microbiology, posted this comparison of the germ theory and Béchamp's cellular theory, which suggests it is conditions within our body that cause disease:

In Pasteur's lifetime there were two competing theories of disease. Evidence is mounting on the side of the cellular theory of disease. The Germ Theory has not been able to help us be healthy.

Germ Theory (Pasteur)

1. Disease arises from microorganisms outside the body.
2. Microorganisms are generally to be guarded against.
3. The function of microorganisms is constant.
4. The shapes and colours of microorganisms are constant.
5. Every disease is associated with a particular microorganism.
6. Microorganisms are primary causal agents.
7. Disease can "strike" anybody.
8. To prevent disease we have to "build defences."

Cellular Theory (Bechamp)

1. Disease arises from microorganisms within the cells of the body.
2. These intracellular microorganisms normally function to build and assist in the metabolic processes of the body.
3. The function of these organisms changes to assist in the catabolic (disintegration) processes of the host organism when that organism dies or is injured, which may be chemical as well as mechanical.
4. Microrganisms change their shapes and colours to reflect the medium.
5. Every disease is associated with a particular condition.
6. Microorganisms become "pathogenic" as the health of the host organism deteriorates. Hence, the condition of the host organism is the primary causal agent.
7. Disease is built by unhealthy conditions.
8. To prevent disease we have to create health.

When I choose what to eat, I don't wonder if it contains "pathogens." I really can't tell for sure if it does. What matters is that the food will make me healthier. To know this, I have to know where it came from, how it was produced, did the people producing it enjoy what they were doing? How did the food make me feel the last time I ate it?

If you believe in the germ theory of disease, you are dependent on scientists and government agencies to test and certify your food safe. The cellular theory gives you control and responsibility for maintaining your own health by choosing food that builds a healthy system.

Everyone has to find the way to eat that best suits them.

I feel the best when most of my calories come from fats like butter, cream, cheese, nuts, marrow from bones and eggs. All from animals raised on pasture without any grain. Fresh or fermented fruits and vegetables along with this is enough. Processed foods aren't good and cooked food is not as good as raw food. Probiotics in the form of kefir is the one thing I always eat every day.[21]

That this debate is happening in the early 2000s isn't just a random occurrence.

Just when it looked as if our government had finally gotten rid of raw milk, and of infectious disease, both began to reappear. A hard core of consumers, especially in California, where retail sales have long been legal, continued drinking it, but the numbers have expanded significantly, to the point that, by 2006 and 2007, Sally Fallon Morell of the Weston A. Price Foundation estimated there were at least half a million American consumers. Some public health officials I heard speak on the subject estimated that possibly one percent or more of the population drink raw milk; that would translate into three million or more consumers.

By the early 2000s, we had big problems with two pathogens. There was *E. coli* O157:H7, which was first discovered in 1982, apparently developing in feedlots as a mutation of normally harmless strains of *E. coli* bacteria.[22] It was infecting all kinds of foods, from fresh spinach to hamburger meat to fast food tacos. Then there was something called MRSA (methicillin-resistant *Staphylococcus aureus*)—bacterial infections resistant to most of our antibiotics. Studies showed that by 2005, more people were dying from MRSA than AIDS, and a study in the *Journal of the American Medical Association* called it "a major public health problem" that had moved from primarily infecting hospital patients to hitting the population at large in places like health clubs and school gyms.[23]

It got so that scientists began expressing concern that maybe we were overdoing it in our germ-fighting efforts, such as by making anti-bacterial soaps much more widely available in homes, offices, schools, and health clubs.

A Tufts University analysis published in the journal *Emerging Infectious Diseases* stated, "Scientists are concerned that the antibacterial agents will select bacteria resistant to them and cross-resistant to antibiotics. Moreover, if they alter a person's microflora, they may negatively affect the normal maturation of the T helper cell response of the immune system to commensal flora antigens; this change could lead to a greater chance of allergies in children."[24]

In the view of raw milk advocates like Mark McAfee, owner of Organic Pastures Dairy Co., we have come full circle as a society. Milk pasteurization had the effect of beginning a trend toward removing active beneficial bacteria and enzymes from our food—bacteria and enzymes that help strengthen our immune systems and thereby protect us from pathogens and the chronic disease that results from deficiencies in our systems. The Organic Pastures Web site explains it this way:

> More and more US consumers have severely weakened immune systems and can become ill by eating small amounts of foreign bacteria that their bodies are not familiar with. It has been estimated that about 70% of the strength of a healthy immune system is made up of the diversity of living bacteria found in the intestines. Raw milk provides a perfect source for the "seeding and feeding" of these diverse populations of living bacteria. The average American diet is practically devoid of living bacteria (all killed foods and few bacterial sources). Our immune systems have suffered as a direct result. Consuming raw milk and dairy products is an important step towards regaining immune strength and overall health.[25]

What McAfee is suggesting in his assessment—that "the average American diet is practically devoid of living bacteria"—is that the triumph of the germ theory has changed America's attitudes toward its food and external environment in profound ways. Instead of seeing ourselves as coexisting with bacteria, we see ourselves in battle with them. Moreover, rather than viewing bacteria as diverse living organisms, we have come to see them as monolithic, in a negative way. In a sense, we are at war with bacteria, and that war plays itself out in many strange and convoluted ways, as we'll see in the next chapter.

CHAPTER FOUR

Picking Up the Pieces

What had essentially happened in Michigan, Ohio, and California is that government regulators moved forcefully, in near unison, to clamp down on dairy farmers suspected of selling bad milk. Then, surprise, it turned out that there were doubts about whether raw milk really made the victims sick.

What did the authorities do in the face of such uncertainty? They did what politicians do whenever the immediate cause of a war turns out to be different from what they suspected (or envisioned)—they continued the fight as aggressively as ever.

The likelihood that North Vietnamese gunboats didn't fire on American warships in the Gulf of Tonkin in 1965 didn't cause us to cancel the Vietnam War any more than the fact that we never found weapons of mass destruction caused us to end the Iraq war, some forty years later. And so it was in the raw milk war, which began in 2006. Government health authorities took very different approaches in each of these three places, but the intended effect was the same: to clamp down on the availability of raw milk.

Indeed, one thing that quickly became apparent to me in following up on the cases against raw milk producers in Michigan, Ohio, and California was that local officials had no interest in the germ theory—or any other scientific theory, for that matter. These cases had moved from the public health and law enforcement arenas to the legal and political spheres. In those arenas, the issues, from the viewpoint of the authorities, were narrow and specific, having to do with highly technical and often arcane dairy, agriculture, and food laws and regulations. Political considerations, driven by public sentiments, often affect how intensively the legal issues are pushed.

And what of the illnesses that had triggered this official interest in raw milk producers? They were seemingly forgotten . . . or were they?

Once you enter the legal and political arenas, of course, the process slows down a great deal. What this slowdown meant for the farmers and raw milk consumers in Michigan, Ohio, and California was that, on the surface, things seemingly returned to the way they had been before the authorities intervened.

By late 2006, Richard Hebron went back to servicing food co-ops in Michigan and Illinois. His computer was still being held by authorities as "evidence," but a friend eventually loaned him one as a replacement.

In Ohio, Gary Oaks was on his way to recovering from his terror-filled afternoon in a Cincinnati parking lot, and the only obvious difference in his raw milk herd-share operation was that members had to cross the nearby border into Kentucky to fetch their milk themselves, instead of having Gary deliver it. Near Dayton, Carol Schmitmeyer was back to caring for her hundred cows and her five children, and providing milk to her 150 shareholders.

And in California's vast Central Valley, Mark McAfee returned to supplying the three-hundred-plus retail stores across the state and visiting dozens of farmer's markets, selling raw milk, cream, butter, kefir, and other raw dairy products to his thirty-thousand-plus weekly customers.

However, for the regulators and prosecutors involved in these cases, the wheels of justice were only beginning to turn. Because the American system of government is still highly decentralized, each locale's approach to handling its raw milk crisis was different.

Yet despite the decentralization, Washington's influence has grown in the area of public health, as it has in nearly every area of our lives. So the FDA's influence was an important factor overlaying each of these situations. Because the FDA and the state agricultural agencies generally make their decisions in great secrecy, it's difficult to know exactly how pronounced was the cooperation among federal and state agencies. But as will become clear in the description that follows, cooperation against raw milk is routine.

Michigan: The Law's Long Tentacles

The post-raid atmosphere was probably more highly charged in Michigan than in California or Ohio. The head of the Michigan Department of Agriculture's Food and Dairy Division, Katherine Fedder, had, after all, expended considerable resources organizing the sting against Richard Hebron. An undercover agent had been assigned to infiltrate the co-op, state police were ordered to track Richard Hebron's movements delivering milk to the co-op, and a state court was petitioned to issue search warrants.

After the raid, there was a hue and cry from co-op members and other consumers, some of whom expressed their outrage to the politicians. Chris Kolb, at the time a Democratic member of the Michigan House of Representatives, representing the Ann Arbor area, told me his office had received "a lot" of complaints, and he was siding with the consumers. "There is a demand, there is a supply, so why are we getting in the way of this? . . . People have been drinking raw milk forever."

The office of Michigan's senior US senator, Carl Levin, also received complaints—enough so that he penned a letter of complaint to the US Food and Drug Administration noting that "the cow-share agreement is a private contract where FFC members paid for the boarding, care, and milking of a cow that produces raw milk." He wondered whether the FDA had previously investigated cow-share arrangements, and concluded by questioning whether there were "provisions under FDA regulations that allow citizens to purchase and consume raw milk."

And while things seemed to return to normal for Richard Hebron, in that he continued to make dairy deliveries, in fact his business life had become considerably more difficult. He lost his Ann Arbor distribution outlet at Morgan & York. Fortunately for him, several co-op members arranged for him to use a member's barn for making his Friday deliveries. He had to make similar arrangements to cover two other drop-off points around Detroit and three in Illinois, which suddenly became unavailable because of the publicity surrounding his case.

All the publicity also scared some of his shareholders away. Apparently some consumers figured that if Richard could be hauled off for distributing raw milk, they could similarly get into trouble with the law for drinking it. He concluded that he lost up to a quarter of his business in the weeks following the seizure.

It's difficult to overstate the pall of fear and suspicion that was cast over the life of Richard Hebron. When he resumed deliveries two weeks after the confiscation of his products in mid-October, one Ann Arbor co-op member posted a five-by-ten-foot sign in the new barn drop-off point: THIS COULD BE OUR LAST DELIVERY. The sign urged people to write the MDA and FDA and protest.

When I learned that Hebron had found a new Ann Arbor distribution site, I held off writing about it on my blog, and only after the fact explained that I hadn't revealed the information for fear that the authorities might order another raid—a raid I didn't want to be inadvertently responsible for having triggered.

To Katherine Fedder of the MDA, though, consumer sentiments were irrelevant. This was a matter of laws and regulations and, in her view, Richard Hebron had violated possibly two different laws: Michigan's Grade A Milk Law and the Michigan Food Law of 2000. "We have requirements for what can be sold and what cannot be sold," she told me.

An MDA Food and Dairy Division newsletter from 2002 explains the state's dairy law this way: "Only pasteurized milk and milk products shall be offered for sale or sold, directly or indirectly, to the final consumer. . . . While Michigan law does not prohibit dairy farmers from drinking the raw milk they produce on their farms, MDA strongly advises against this practice." The newsletter also notes proudly that Michigan was the first state during the late 1940s to make pasteurization mandatory.[1]

The Food Law of 2000 prohibits "the misbranding, adulteration, manufacture, distribution, and sale of foods in violation of this act . . ." according to a legislative summary. Of course, if a particular food is banned from sale, then it can't be available at a grocery store. And if it's banned *and* not fully labeled (with quantity, dates, et cetera), well, that's a double whammy. In Fedder's view, the distribution of raw milk from the Morgan & York supply shed was a clear violation of both the dairy law and the food law.[2]

To members of the Family Farms Co-op and its supporters, the MDA newsletter's statement that "Michigan law does not prohibit dairy farmers from drinking the raw milk they produce on their farms" was key. The co-op members, through their herd-share agreement with Richard Hebron, were legally part owners of the cows whose milk they drank—in their view, they were no different from the farmers whom the MDA said were allowed to consume raw milk.

According to then-representative Kolb, "I'm not aware of anything that would rule out owning a share of a cow. As far as I know, you can't sell to the general public. But a farmer can drink raw milk. So if you are an owner of a cow, you can. . . . It's an extension of that."

But Fedder wasn't buying the argument. To her, the consumers were paying for the milk, and therefore they were buying it.

While the MDA could hand out cease-and-desist orders to retailers, as it did to Morgan & York to prevent it from allowing its storage area to be used in distribution of raw milk to co-op members, it couldn't actually prosecute farmers for alleged violations of state laws. In Michigan, that was up to elected county prosecutors. So Fedder put together her evidence and handed it over to the prosecuting attorney in Cass County, the area in western Michigan where Richard Hebron lived.

The prosecutor there was forty-nine-year-old Victor Fitz, a tall, handsome man very much in the mold of the prosecutors we tend to see in television legal and detective dramas. Fitz was in a different position than Fedder. For one thing, he didn't know much about agriculture, since he didn't go after many farmers—most of his cases involved drugs and homicides. And because he was an elected official, he was more inclined to prosecute cases that outraged the community, and less inclined to prosecute those that didn't. Was the distribution of unpasteurized milk in the former or latter category?

I wanted to keep up with the case for my blog, and so I telephoned Fitz every three or four weeks to see how the case was progressing. He initially seemed to think the case was pretty straightforward. In late October, he told me he expected to receive the last of the evidence and reports within a couple of weeks, and to have a decision about whether to prosecute the case a week after that.

As November stretched into December and then into January 2007, it was obvious Fitz hadn't anticipated just how involved this case really was. I knew of one complication—the fact that Richard Hebron had been acquiring the co-op's milk from an Amish farmer just across the state border, in Indiana. Richard told me early on, when I interviewed him about the case, that the farmer had requested that his identity be kept confidential.

The Amish farmer was right to be concerned. Federal law, reinforced by a 1987 court decision, prohibits the interstate shipment of unpasteurized milk not destined for pasteurization.

By early 2007, as I kept up with Victor Fitz, I learned that his investigative tentacles had extended not only to Indiana and the Amish farmer, but clear out to Pennsylvania. While Fitz was willing to take most of my calls, he was quite circumspect in what he told me, being careful not to provide many details. He obviously wanted to keep the channels of communication open with me as a media person, but didn't want me to know specifics of his investigation.

In early February, I learned from attorney Pete Kennedy of Sarasota, Florida, that the Amish farmer was finally ready to go public. (Kennedy worked for the Weston A. Price Foundation, advising farmers, like Richard Hebron, who were in trouble with the law.) I arranged a telephone interview and had a lengthy conversation with David Hochstetler, the forty-eight-year-old farmer whose seventy cows supplied the Family Farms Co-op with raw milk.

It turned out that, within a week of the MDA's sting operation in October 2006, Hochstetler had been visited by several FDA agents looking around his farm and asking questions about what he did with his milk. "I told them this is not in their jurisdiction and that this lease program is not interstate commerce," he recalled. "We had no idea what was going to happen next."

What happened next was that in January 2007, he received the dreaded "warning letter." This is a letter in which the FDA identifies what it sees as violations—in this case, shipping raw milk across state lines—and demands that the recipient correct the problem, under threat of further legal action, including a court-ordered shutdown of the farm.

Hochstetler, who has eight children, told me he was both disgusted and stressed out. "It's politics. It's not a healthy-food issue. It's big agribusiness and the pharmaceutical companies behind this. All they're interested in is protecting the money in their pockets. They don't care about healthy food."

As for the stress, it was "something that is on your mind all day long. . . . It's hard to concentrate on the things we should concentrate on."

But Hochstetler said he was determined to "continue on" his path of supplying raw milk to consumers who wanted it so badly. He described for me how he and his twenty-year-old son had gone together to help deliver milk to consumers in the Chicago area. "They thank us from the bottom of their hearts," he said. "A lot of mothers say how their children had asthma and allergies and they tried everything the medical profession had to offer and nothing worked until they tried raw milk. There was even a man whose wife has multiple sclerosis. He said that every time she drinks raw milk, she feels stronger. He said, 'This is all I've got.'"

A number of Family Farm Co-op members voiced support via letters. One of them even went so far as to offer legal assistance. Steve Bemis, then a pension lawyer with a major corporation, accompanied Hochstetler to the FDA Detroit regional office to plead for a rescinding of the warning letter. In addition to the four FDA Detroit officials present, an FDA official from Indianapolis and another from the agency's headquarters in Rockville, Maryland, joined in via phone.

Bemis says he argued to the FDA officials that for farmers, confusion exists as to whether the FDA's rule prohibiting interstate commerce of raw milk applies to cow-share arrangements. He also pointed out that Hochstetler had previously informed state officials about his involvement in a cow-share arrangement. The fact that no government officials followed up before the October 13 sting operation could be interpreted as tacit approval, he said.

The FDA acceded to a request from Bemis to give Hochstetler an extension of fifteen days to file a written response to the warning letter. Big sports.

Pete Kennedy also put me in touch with the Pennsylvania farmer who was being investigated by Fitz: Wilmer Newswanger, a Mennonite whose farm was about thirty miles west of the capital city of Harrisburg. A friendly man, Newswanger told me he had been supplying cheeses—Cheddar, Monterey Jack, Colby, baby Swiss, Gouda, and Havarti—to the Family Farms Cooperative. They were made from raw milk, but aged the sixty days required by the FDA before they could legally be sold via retail. (The sixty-day rule for aging raw milk cheese allows for the fact that cheese over that period of aging essentially "self-pasteurizes" in terms of destroying any potentially harmful pathogens.)

Newswanger described for me two visits he had had from agents. The first, in early December, was from agents of the Pennsylvania Department of Agriculture. "They mentioned product going to Michigan," Newswanger recalled. "And they had questions about Richard Hebron." They looked through his UPS shipments for the previous three weeks.

Then, just before Christmas, he had a visit from agents from the FDA. They also had questions about his relationship with Richard Hebron, as well as about his procedures for producing cheese.

In March 2007, I had the good fortune to meet Richard Hebron while I was traveling on business in Michigan. A reader of my blog, Linda Diane Feldt, an Ann Arbor holistic practitioner, hosted a potluck dinner at her home. Several dozen members of the Family Farms Co-op were there, and Hebron made the trip as well, to thank everyone for their support. He told me his computer was still being held as evidence, and he had no idea when Victor Fitz, the Cass County prosecutor, would make a decision on his case. While some of the Ann Arbor herd-share members were coming back on board—in part because they missed the health benefits of their raw milk— Hebron's business wasn't back to where it was before the raid.

What I didn't relate to Hebron at that time was my concern that Fitz was preparing to throw the book at Hebron, based on the fact that the investigation was taking so long and was so far-flung. After all, it only made sense that Fitz would want to justify all the investigative resources he was putting into the case.

Ohio: Legalities Substitute for Illnesses

If you read through the regulatory and legal documents in the case involving dairy farmer Carol Schmitmeyer—the Ohio Department of Agriculture hearing summary, her court appeal, and the judge's decision—you find no mention of the child and elderly man from Dayton who supposedly became ill from drinking her dairy's raw milk. It's the case I described in chapter 1. And the reason is not that authorities forgot about the illnesses.

I spoke with Lewis Jones, chief of the ODA's Dairy Division, in early November 2006, and he told me that the Montgomery County Health Department, which includes Dayton, had concluded, based on "epidemiological" evidence, that raw milk had sickened the boy and the elderly man.

What about the denial by the man and the boy's family, who maintained they were likely made sick by something else—the boy by bird feces in snow he ate and the man by deli meats? Jones had a ready answer: "That's what's so dangerous" about raw milk, he told me. "If people get sick, they'll say it was something else."

Carol Schmitmeyer had further evidence to back up the two consumer claims: She told me that health department inspectors took numerous samples from her dairy's milk, and "They found nothing" in the way of pathogens. "They were trying to make it look like raw milk" had made the two individuals ill.

So apparently the authorities decided not to risk weakening their case, and instead focused on the herd-share arrangement that Carol had established in 2005, to enable her to provide raw milk to 150 consumers without violating Ohio's prohibition on the sale of raw milk.

The tipoff to Schmitmeyer that the assault on her herd-share agreement really stemmed from the reported illnesses was that she had gone to the trouble in 2005 to hire the ODA's former in-house counsel as her lawyer to draw up the herd-share agreement. "We're scratching our heads and wondering why ODA won't tell us what we need to do to make it legal."

Of course, there was nothing she could do to make it legal. The ODA held a hearing in September 2006, presided over by a hearing officer appointed by the ODA. That is typical in such state agency hearings, and it gives you a sense of their impartiality, or lack thereof.

The ODA argued that Carol used the herd-share arrangement as a way to circumvent Ohio's law against the sale of unpasteurized milk, and the hearing officer, a man by the name of Andrew Cooke, agreed. Here is his recommendation:

> During the period up to and including October 2005, Carol Schmitmeyer and her husband distributed raw milk in unlabeled hand-filled jugs at a cost of $6.00 per gallon, without an Ohio milk processor license. Respondent utilized a herd-share agreement to allow her to argue that the raw milk she delivered was not sold but provided to owners of her herd. Respondent's herd-share agreement, however, is nothing more than a thinly veiled attempt to shield Respondent from liability for her illegal sales of raw milk. For this reason, and the reasons stated above, it is recommended that the Ohio Department of Agriculture revoke the Grade A milk producer license of Carol Schmitmeyer.

Schmitmeyer's only hope of overturning the ODA's decision was to go to state court. Even there, in a supposedly impartial setting, the odds were long. Judges are generally reluctant to disagree with government agencies. Their feeling is that the government officials know the regulations and laws better than anyone, and are going to do things by the book. Moreover, because courts are so backed up, simply getting a decision can take months, or even years.

But because of the urgency of the situation, Schmitmeyer's lawyer, Gary Cox, was able to get her case heard sooner than it might otherwise have been. And lo and behold, the judge, Jonathan P. Heine, was listening.[3]

Judge Heine was concerned that the hearing officer had refused to allow Cox to question ODA officials about possible inconsistencies in Ohio's dairy law, whereby farm owners are allowed to consume milk directly from their cows. He wondered, in his opinion: "Does the Department allow herd owners and their children/family members to consume raw milk? Or must the children/family members reside in the farm household? Or must the children/family members also be active participants in the milking operation in order to 'legally' consume raw milk?"

Further, "if the cows are owned by a partnership, can all partners consume raw milk? Or must the partners be family members? Or must the partners consuming the raw milk reside on the farm? And if the cows are owned by a corporation, the same troubling questions apply with even more shareholders being involved in the equation."

The judge provided an answer of sorts to his questions when he stated, "The Department . . . argues that the 'herd-share agreement' is a transparent attempt to circumvent the law. If the herd-share agreement is a circumvention of the law, so is the Department's inexact practice of allowing owners and their families, etc. to consume raw milk."

The judge almost seemed to be having fun with the absurdity of the ODA's failure to distinguish between the farmer/owner herd-share members when he stated: "Under another hypothetical, the Court could define a 'sale' in a way which would allow delivery of raw milk to all persons who have a small or remote interest in a dairy cow, provided the owner consumes the raw milk on the farm. This definition might allow delivery to herd-share owners, but only if the raw milk is consumed on the farm. Numerous other examples could be propounded depending on the practices allowed by the Department."

He scolded the hearing officer for failing to define the terms *sale* and *sold*, especially "given their importance in determining the outcome of this case . . ."

Then he added:

> In the absence of necessary definitions by either the Department or the Legislature, and in view of the Department of Agriculture's policy or practice which permits the use and consumption of raw milk by some undefined class of persons at unspecified locations, the Court is unable to conclude as a matter of law whether or not the Appellant is a raw milk retailer within the context of Chapter 917. Further, the Court is unable to conclude as a matter of law whether the herd-share agreement is "a thinly veiled attempt" to avoid regulation under Chapter 917 as concluded by the hearing officer and the Director of the Department. The Court finds that the decision of the Director of the Department of Agriculture to revoke the Appellant's Grade A milk producer license is not supported by substantial, reliable and probative evidence and that the decision was not in accordance with law.

The decision?

> **IT IS THEREFORE ORDERED AND DECREED** that the appeal by Carol Schmitmeyer is granted and the order to revoke Appellant's Grade A milk producer license as issued by the Director of the Department of Agriculture on September 28, 2006 is vacated.

This decision was a big victory not only for Carol Schmitmeyer, but also for all consumers who looked to the herd-share arrangement as a way to obtain raw milk in states where actual sales were banned. But one question remained: Would the ODA appeal the decision?

California: Setting a Legislative Time Bomb

Once the California Department of Food and Agriculture and public health authorities gave Mark McAfee the all-clear in late September 2006, the way seemed to open for him to resume growing Organic Pastures Dairy Co., his four-hundred-acre Fresno raw dairy. McAfee is a consummate marketer, and to him the shutdown was, perversely, the beginning of "a perfect marketing storm." The more the authorities cracked down on him, the more publicity he received and the faster he grew.

He couldn't have imagined how eager the authorities would be to resume playing the game with him. Because while the CDFA may have left his dairy embarrassed at not having found evidence of *E. coli* O157:H7, it wasn't close to being through with Mark McAfee.

CDFA's branch chief of Milk and Dairy Food Safety, Stephen Beam, had come up with an idea to bring Mark's dairy to its knees. Of course, Beam, a tall, lanky, sandy-haired man, wouldn't publicly admit that that was his objective. But if you look at the record, that's what appears to have occurred.

In mid-October 2006, just two weeks after Organic Pastures Dairy reopened, Beam proposed adding a legal cleanliness standard that would have the effect of tightening California's dairy law—tightening it so much that Organic Pastures might encounter problems meeting it.

Beam didn't tell me the story himself, though he confirmed it when we met briefly at a conference of milk regulators in April 2009. In a court deposition he gave after his scheme became public and a suit was filed against his agency in 2008, Beam explained what happened beginning in the weeks immediately after the CDFA cleared McAfee, and Organic Pastures resumed operations and again began to capitalize on the raw milk boom.

In his testimony, Beam describes a seemingly dry bureaucratic process—how he filled out a form for proposing new legislation

> that basically describes the concept, the background, and then, you know, the pros and cons, and then proposes, you know, text that would speak to whatever amendments or changes or additions that might need to be made. And those come out of the branch. And those go forward from the branch, and they go to our superiors. For example, from me it would go to our division office and then from the division office it would go up to the executive office, and ultimately to the Legislative Affairs Office.

The new legislation sounded harmless enough—it would require that milk from raw dairies not contain more than ten coliforms (a nonpathogenic bacteria common to milk) per milliliter. While coliforms are considered by everyone involved in the milk industry to be harmless to people, there is considerable debate over what their presence signifies as to the cleanliness of milk and the possibility that pathogens could appear, a matter I cover in detail in chapter 11. And because the number of coliforms can vary widely from batch to batch of raw milk, from less than ten to one hundred or more, there is an equal amount of disagreement over whether raw dairies can even consistently meet a ten-coliform-per-milliliter standard on a regular enough basis to remain commercially sustainable. In other words, the new standard could have had the effect of putting Organic Pastures out of business.

Whose idea was it to propose this new legislation? According to Beam's testimony, "The concept originated from my branch, and then I served as a technical resource as the bill went forward. . . . I'm responsible as the chief of the branch for concepts that go forward from the program for consideration within the Department for a legislative idea or concept or proposal."[4]

By early February 2007, Beam said, his two superiors at CDFA—Dr. Annette Whiteford and Dr. Richard Breitmeyer—had approved the proposal and sent it on to the California Assembly's Agriculture Committee. Beam's solo—some might call it secretive—decision to include a ten-coliform-per-milliliter standard was on track to become a hidden time bomb, set to explode in the dynamic cauldron of California food politics.

CHAPTER FIVE

Raw Milk and the Cases of the Disappearing Pathogens

On April 5, 2007, the New York Department of Agriculture and Markets posted two brief press releases—each about 250 words—announcing that Breese Hollow Dairy in Hoosick and Beech Hill Farms in Greenwich had "voluntarily" suspended raw milk sales because their milk had tested positive for *Listeria monocytogenes.*

According to one of the releases, "Listeria contaminated products can cause listeriosis, a disease that can cause mild flu-like symptoms in healthy individuals, and more serious conditions in immune-compromised individuals."

As brief as the press releases were, they were obviously bad news for the dairies involved. They would have been bad news in any day and age, but especially in the Internet age because stories circulate so widely and so rapidly. Anytime someone were to search the Web for "Breese Hollow Dairy" or "Beech Hill Farms" to find information about the dairies—perhaps about the availability of raw milk or to assess which raw milk dairies are likeliest to be safe—those press releases would come up . . . and would continue coming up for years into the future.

I assumed that, because the information was coming from New York, it would likely be more reliable than what I was accustomed to in Michigan and Ohio. New York seemed to have one of the more enlightened approaches to raw milk in the country. Unlike Michigan and Ohio, which simply banned raw milk sales by limiting the market to pasteurized milk, New York allowed dairy farmers who wanted to sell raw milk to obtain a special permit that allowed sales with certain limitations: The milk could only be sold to consumers directly from the farm, and it needed to be tested by the state every thirty days for pathogens. In addition, dairy farmers selling raw milk were limited to selling only fluid milk; no sales of other raw dairy products like cream, butter, and yogurt were allowed. A growing number of dairies were taking advantage of the program—some eighteen had obtained permits by early 2007, compared with twelve a year earlier.

I figured the farmers who ran the dairies cited for listeria would feel badly, as would any food business that has to tell the world the government has raised questions about its product's safety. How had they let the contamination happen?

As things turned out, I wasn't in a position to follow up until two months later, in June. By that time I encountered two very upset farmers—but they were upset for different reasons than I expected.

David "Chuck" Phippen, the owner of Breese Hollow Dairy, was obviously angry when I caught him on the phone. He had thirty cows and had been selling raw milk for two years from his farm, following eleven years of selling milk commercially for pasteurization. "We know we have a good product. We've never had a problem" with customers becoming ill, he told me.

Phippen was also upset that he had been fined $300 by the New York Department of Agriculture and Markets. "I have to sell a lot of milk to make back that $300," he said. "I have ten kids. I can't hire high-powered attorneys" to fight the state's contention.

Well, I inquired, you may be upset, but did you or did you not have *Listeria monocytogenes* in your milk? "They said they test the milk and that one cell of listeria amounts to contamination. They said we adulterated the milk. They refused to re-test the milk [that is, the same milk in which the listeria was discovered]. When they tested our milk two weeks later, it was okay."

Next I telephoned Dawn Sharts, the owner of Beech Hill Farms. I discovered that she was, if anything, angrier than Phippen. "They treat us like criminals, like we are selling toxic waste," she told me.

What especially bothered this fifty-three-year-old farmer was that she'd had such high hopes for her dairy's raw milk sales. The possibility of an additional product that could generate significant additional cash was compelling. After filling out a bunch of forms and spending more than $1,000 to have her cows tested for bovine tuberculosis and other diseases, she passed inspections and received her permit in January 2006.

"I was excited. This was going to be a new product line for us," Sharts explained. She had been steadily receiving more requests for unpasteurized milk from consumers who would call, e-mail, and stop in at her Greenwich farm. Especially exciting to her was the fact that she could collect $6 a gallon from customers coming to the farm to buy raw milk, versus the $2 or so she was receiving from local processors who pasteurized her milk for sale in grocery stores.

She also liked the idea that the state would be testing her milk regularly, providing reassurance to customers that her product was as pure as she felt it to be. Within weeks of receiving her permit, she had a dozen customers regularly visiting the farm to purchase raw milk. Word about a new raw milk outlet gets around quickly.

But before long, there were signs of trouble as well. There were wide discrepancies in readings of somatic cell counts—routine measurements of white blood cells that are required of all milk, including that intended for pasteurization, and used in the industry as an indication of overall milk cleanliness. A reading of less than one hundred thousand is considered excellent. Sharts said the state in early March 2006 came up with a reading of 550,000, while the processor that handles the dairy's milk intended for pasteurization came up with a reading of only 55,000 on the same day's milk.

The test that had led to the listeria finding was suspicious as well. Both her dairy and Phippen's were tested on March 26. "To have two farms so far apart [more than twenty miles] and have the same pathogen show up in the tests is not a coincidence," Sharts told me.

In an e-mail to the agriculture department on April 9, she let her feelings hang out:

> You may think I am in denial; however, I do not believe the Listeria was in our milk. I think that it could have been in the test vial taken to the lab, or for that matter it could have happened in the lab itself (as Listeria is everywhere, as everyone agrees) . . . the lab is not in a vacuum, and with all the testing done from across the state [it] is a haven of bacteria. There have been far too many lab problems with me in such a short amount of time to not question their methods. Humans make a lot of mistakes. I took microbiology in college and know it is not a perfect science . . .
>
> This whole thing has made me quite upset and sick to my stomach, as you well know. It has been dehumanizing, demoralizing and embarrassing. We try to work so hard at this end to do everything right. This is the way we are treated . . . I alerted my few customers and that was all that needed to be done. I believe that the monetary penalty is outrageous and unfair, especially since the pathogen is

everywhere and I have no control as to how it got into the sample. If I were responsible for something that would cause the public to get sick because I was a sloppy farmer, then I could understand the penalty.

The press release is another outrageous and unfair practice, as I know the only reason to do it is to cover your bottoms. Farmers get enough bad press. No one is going to get sick, and actually you people should follow up with a press release after the subsequent test . . . [reporting] that the milk is fine. I know you people will not do that because you do not want me selling raw milk and therefore by putting that in the paper would only support raw milk sales. All of this has been to try and scare me. Well, I am not afraid of the government nor do I trust the government, and this just gives me more reason not to.

Sharts didn't limit herself to writing e-mails. To support her claim that the agriculture inspectors were careless in conducting their inspections, and thus might inadvertently have introduced *Listeria monocytogenes* into the milk, she had her son mount video cameras in the milking parlor.

She wanted to see if the camera could catch the inspectors unnecessarily opening her bulk tank (exposing the milk to contamination) and failing to properly clean their boots and hands. When the inspectors came on April 13 to reinspect her dairy, she had the camera rolling. She put the video onto the Internet, and I linked to it in an article I wrote about Sharts for BusinessWeek.com.[1]

In one segment, an inspector can be seen opening the bulk tank and looking in; in a second segment, an inspector is shown rolling up her pants after having been in the barnyard with chickens and other animals, thus possibly contaminating her hands.

What did New York's Department of Agriculture and Markets have to say to the charges from Phippen and Sharts that the testing for *Listeria monocytogenes* was unfair? Not a lot. When I asked if the state's lab had had any misreadings, spokesperson Jessica Chittenden said, "We are not aware of any misreadings at the State Food Lab."

How about the coincidence of both farms being more than twenty miles apart, and measuring bad for listeria on the same day?

"The State Food Lab did genetically fingerprint the isolates from the two farms' samples and found the two samples to contain two different strains of listeria," she said. "We realized the concern [the coincidence] raised. To clear things up, we ran the genetic fingerprint test."

Such a test had helped agriculture officials in California determine that the *E. coli* O157:H7 that sickened spinach consumers was different from the one that allegedly sickened six children in the state the previous September (though the *E. coli* wasn't found in the raw milk the authorities concluded had been responsible for the illnesses).

But in New York, might the differences in the genetic makeup of the two examples of listeria possibly have been attributable to careless inspector techniques, carelessness that could have lead to different strains of *Listeria monocytogenes* being brought into the two barns? In other words, might the listeria found in each dairy's milk have originated in the barnyard at each of the two farms?

Nothing doing, argued the agriculture department's spokesperson.

> All inspection staff and laboratory staff follow standard FDA protocol for sampling and testing milk. They are trained and evaluated every three years. Examples of procedures include: samples from bulk tanks are taken from openings in the top of the tank, not from the outlet valve or spout where it can be easily contaminated. Gloves are not routinely worn when taking samples; instead hands are thoroughly washed. Sterile vials are always used. They are purchased sterile and dipped in sanitizer before being filled as an extra precaution. Boots are also washed and sanitized, more as an animal disease preventative measure than a milk quality issue. Controls exist in the lab to detect cross-contamination, an event that has never occurred on any samples tested for listeria.

In other words, the department was saying, despite the lapses Dawn Sharts's video might have shown, there was no way the department could have screwed up.

I had one other question of the department: Had anyone become ill from the contaminated milk? After all, the test results came back at least two weeks after the farm had sold the milk, meaning that most or all had been consumed. "Not that we are aware of," said Chittenden.

In the weeks following the issuance of the April 5 press release announcing the presence of listeria in her milk, Sharts figured she heard from "at least half a dozen people. They said they are thrilled they can get raw milk. Chuck

Phippen and I are the only ones in this area that have it. I had a woman call from Salem, three or four miles from here. She said, 'I heard about the listeria problem and I'm interested in buying raw milk.' She wanted to know when she could come by and pick it up.'"

But alas, Sharts had to tell everyone to go to Phippen's farm instead. Even though Sharts's milk was found to be free of pathogens in that subsequent test in early April she videotaped, Sharts had decided to exit the raw milk business.

"An inspector told me, 'New York State doesn't want you to be able to sell raw milk,'" she said. "It's not so much a financial hardship for us [to endure such harassment] as the insult from the state. It was embarrassing to see our name out there. Our farm is very clean. It makes us feel sick to our stomachs to see what they have put us through." In early May 2007, she sent her raw milk permit back to New York's Department of Agriculture and Markets.

This theme, of milk supposedly contaminated by *Listeria monocytogenes*, would come up again and again. In early August, I heard from a third New York farmer, Lori McGrath, who with her husband, Darren, owns Autumn Valley Farm in Worcester, New York. Here's how I started the report of Lori on my blog:[2]

> The press release about listeria contamination of the farm's raw milk has been posted online and sent to local newspapers. The calls have gone out to the three customers who purchased the milk, warning them to dispose of it. The farm has "voluntarily suspended" raw milk sales. Within a few weeks, New York's Department of Agriculture & Markets can be expected to impose a $300 fine on the farmer.
>
> But this, the fourth New York state raw milk dairy to test positive [another farmer, Jerry Snyder, owner of Sunny Cove Farm in Alfred, New York, had tested positive a few months earlier) for *Listeria monocytogenes* in the last eight months (a fifth was cited for campylobacter), vows not to just be another statistic.
>
> Lori McGrath, owner with her husband, Darren, of Autumn Valley Farm in Worcester, New York, vows to fight back. "I don't intend on letting them bully us."
>
> Lori and her husband have operated the 160-acre dairy for six years, and have had their raw milk license for eight months. "We gave up our entire (professional) lives six years ago to be farmers. . . . We worked too hard to let them take this away."

Like many raw-milk producers and consumers alike, Lori wonders why no one has become ill from the supposed pathogens. She also wonders why the state isn't investigating the problem further. "You'd think they'd wonder if there's an epidemic," since so many cows are turning out milk with *Listeria monocytogenes*.

Lori feels the state is simply trying to sow fear, based on its own fears. "The raw milk demand is exploding, and they don't know what to do about it."

New York's raw-milk dairy farmers are clearly becoming tired of what they consider to be government harassment. If Lori McGrath is any indication, not only are they becoming tired, they're not going to take it any more.

It's easy to appreciate these farmers' anger. Farming is hard work, requiring grueling days of feeding animals, shoveling manure, attaching and unattaching milking equipment, fixing damaged fencing, herding stubborn cows, being on hand at all hours of the night for new calf births, and so on and so forth. And because cows have to be milked twice a day, 365 days a year, you can't take time off without finding replacement labor to do the milking and animal maintenance.

It's financially quite risky as well. Lori told me that she and Darren left a regular work life to buy their dairy farm in 2001, because he "has always had this passion for farming." One of their first steps was to rip out the existing milking parlor and replace it with one they designed themselves, with equipment they imported from New Zealand. They committed to a natural type of dairy farming, avoiding grain feeding and instead letting their forty-four cows graze during spring and summer, and feeding them hay in winter— all to bolster the milk's nutritional benefits. "It's very labor-intensive," Lori admits.

On top of that, to make ends meet and help pay the cost of having three children in college, Lori continued with a job she had outside the farm, managing a physical therapist's office. That meant she had to live off the farm in the New York City area for three or four days a week.

When they first arrived in Worcester, there were about ten other conventional dairy farms within a few miles of theirs. By the summer of 2007, when she and Darren had to suspend sales because of the listeria finding, the other farms had disappeared, and their owners had taken regular nonfarm jobs, she says.

The couple had received its raw milk license only eight months before the listeria incident. Like Dawn Sharts, they saw raw milk as a way to increase revenues over what they received by selling milk in bulk to processors. And over this eight-month period, they had made progress as they increased their raw milk customer base, reducing the amount of milk sold in bulk to about half of what they produced, down from around 75 percent when they first obtained their raw milk permit.

As in the cases of Chuck Phippen and Dawn Sharts (and Jerry Snyder), no one became ill from the supposedly tainted milk.

The whole experience encouraged Lori McGrath to investigate the problem of *Listeria monocytogenes,* and what she learned surprised her. For one thing, she says she discovered that some labs come back with test results in three days, while the state was taking two weeks. "If they are so concerned about people getting sick, why don't they get the results more quickly?"

She also found that "it's possible to get false positives where there are nonviable listeria cells, really dead cells. *Listeria monocytogenes* cells are difficult to find. It takes a trained eye to even find them."

Perhaps most telling, Lori says she was told by lab experts that "*Listeria monocytogenes* is not found in raw milk, and no one has gotten sick." The state, she argued, "is crying wolf so many times that no one believes them."

The next month, September 2007, the situation became even more bizarre, as the listeria "epidemic" seemed to have spread to California. There, nearly a year to the day following the California Department of Agriculture's shutdown of Organic Pastures (described in chapter 2) in connection with an outbreak of *E. coli* O157:H7, the CDFA announced that it had discovered *Listeria monocytogenes* in cream from Mark McAfee's Organic Pastures Dairy.

In a press release suggesting a serious situation, CDFA stated it had "issued an order to Organic Pastures Dairy Company to withdraw from retail distribution Grade A raw cream manufactured at their facility in Fresno, due to detection of *Listeria monocytogenes* bacteria."

> Under the recall, Organic Pastures brand Grade A raw cream with code dates SEP 14 through SEP 21 is to be pulled immediately from retail shelves and consumers are strongly urged to dispose of any product remaining in their refrigerators. Until further notice, Organic Pastures may not produce raw cream for the retail market.
>
> The quarantine order came following laboratory confirmation

of *Listeria monocytogenes* bacteria. CDFA inspectors found the bacteria as a result of product testing conducted as part of routine inspection and sample collection at the facility.

The withdrawal order involves removal of raw cream from grocery stores, retail outlets and farmers markets throughout California.

The great majority of cream consumed in California is pasteurized. Raw cream is not. Pasteurization eliminates the risk of bacterial illness . . .[3]

Mark McAfee's reaction was similar to that of the New York dairy farmers—he was outraged. "After nine days of testing a sample, they got a positive reading," he told me. He said he was told by a state lab official that the finding "was considered to be subclinical." He said technicians "put the milk in a petri dish and use a special broth that suppresses the growth of other bacteria to encourage the growth of the listeria. By definition, the listeria they get is an extremely low level."[4]

The recall order applied to two hundred pints of cream sent to forty-five stores, out of three hundred stores that normally carry Organic Pastures products. Nearly all the cream had already been purchased, he said; as in New York State, no one had become ill from consuming the product.

My description of the new *Listeria monocytogenes* discovery in California stirred up amazingly strong emotions among bloggers. The incident triggered bad memories for Mary McGonigle-Martin, the mother of one of the children who had become ill the previous September:

> It was an eerie Labor Day weekend here in California. It was blazing hot just like last year. I couldn't help but think about all the people drinking raw milk produced in this heat. Are they vulnerable because it is so hot? Bacteria explode in the heat. I kept wondering, "Is there going to be another outbreak?" I'm glad to hear that so far no one has become ill and I do hope it is a "testing" flaw and not a real contamination problem.
>
> Tomorrow it will be a year since we were told that Chris had a chance of dying simply because of ingesting a food-borne pathogen.

Mary's emotional reaction prompted dozens of other comments in support of Mark McAfee, and questioning CDFA's findings.

Steve Bemis, a Michigan lawyer, a member of the Ann Arbor cooperative served by Richard Hebron, and a board member of the Farm-to-Consumer Legal Defense Fund, observed,

> This epidemic of state testings for **Listeria m.** has the sticky fingerprints of a coordinated campaign all over it. It's an epidemic of testing only, obviously, since I'm aware of no illnesses surrounding any of the situations in Pennsylvania, New York, and now California.

Dave Milano, a part-time farmer in Pennsylvania, expressed concern that

> our blind focus on killing bugs to produce health has hurt us, badly, by diminishing our immunity, and making us MORE susceptible to disease.
>
> Again, no reasonable person is suggesting that grossly dirty food should be tolerated. Sensible steps to maintain cleanliness are welcome and necessary. But obsessive, bacteriophobic hygiene, and its kin, distrust of natural products, are truly dangerous.

Mark McAfee joined the debate, writing:

> Health is about the strength of the immune system. Not about bugs. That is why pathogens do not make 99% of healthy people sick. Find a subclinical level of listeria in some raw cream and nobody is sick and this is news??? . . . The bacteria phobia in our country is beyond stupid. It is causing the sheepeople in this country to eat sterilized foods and further depress their immune systems. Pathogens can only be pathogens if the host is weak. Does anyone get that???? That is why the list of pathogens gets longer and longer. It is because we are weaker and weaker.

Governmental involvement in this matter wasn't over, though, and it would make a bizarre situation totally ridiculous.

Because Organic Pastures was shipping raw dairy products out of state as well, to mail-order customers, the FDA determined it needed to issue its own press release, apparently to warn consumers in other parts of the country about the danger. For reasons that will likely remain forever unknown, several FDA officials asked Mark McAfee to help in writing a press release about the finding. This was a little like asking the fox to keep an eye on things inside the chicken coop.

Ironically, this request from FDA came just as the controversy about Organic Pastures' latest tussle with California's Department of Food and Agriculture had seemingly blown over. McAfee had completed his recall of raw cream the agency warned was contaminated with listeria. CDFA followed up by giving Mark the go-ahead to resume raw cream sales.

Then, out of nowhere, the FDA stuck its nose in and ignited an entirely new chapter in the affair. The problems started when the FDA offered McAfee a chance to put together an initial draft of a press release to be issued by the FDA alerting consumers that twenty-one pints of Organic Pastures raw cream shipped outside of California as "pet food" were part of the original recall ordered by CDFA. If I hadn't seen the e-mail correspondence myself, I would have said that the whole idea of the FDA asking Mark to write a press release was better suited to a *Saturday Night Live* skit than anything that might happen in real life.

Interestingly, McAfee agreed to try his hand at writing a release, and, even more interesting, the release Mark put together started out pretty reasonably (from the FDA's vantage point): "During routine OPDC product tests performed by the State of California at the CDFA lab in Los Angeles, *Listeria monocytogenes* was found." So far, so good.

McAfee then warmed up a bit when he stated, "*Listeria monocytogenes* generally does not cause illness in healthy people unless the consumer is very immune-depressed. Common signs of illness include sepsis and meningitis. *Listeria monocytogenes* is associated with miscarriage of early pregnancy. About 10% of the population carries this pathogen in their intestines and is immune to its effects." Still passable, if you're an FDAer.

But then McAfee really got going: "People that drink raw milk or raw cream on a regular basis have a much stronger and different immune system. This is because of the constant exposure to a broad range of good bacteria not generally found in the standard diet of Americans today."

Needless to say, McAfee's career as an FDA press release writer was short-lived. In an e-mail, Jolene Hedgecock of the FDA's "Recall Team" in San Francisco, wrote:

> FDA does not feel that your suggested draft of the press release is adequate. FDA plans on issuing its own press release (see attached) warning consumers about the raw cream and the raw butter, which

> was made from the raw cream. This is obviously a separate action
> from the decisions made by the State of California. FDA will post
> its press release on the FDA website and issue it to the Associated
> Press. Therefore, FDA feels there is no longer a need for you to issue
> a separate press release.

The FDA version said the FDA "is warning consumers not to drink or
consume foods made from raw cream labeled as 'Organic Pastures Grade A
Raw Cream'" and added, "Consumers are also warned to not consume foods
made from raw butter" from Organic Pastures. And it actually noted, "No
illnesses have been reported to date."

As one might expect, McAfee cared about as much for the FDA's version
as the agency cared for his, except McAfee was more outspoken about his
dissatisfaction. "The bacterial analysis of the raw butter showed no signs of
listeria," he wrote back to Hedgecock. "All tests are negative. In fact, CDFA
official test reports on the raw butter were negative (9-18-07). FDA is warning people not to consume raw butter that has been cleared for sale. Your
proposed FDA press release is factually incorrect and highly misleading.
Adding a warning about raw butter is slanderous and baseless." It all "proves
the FDA intent to slander and express its deep anti-raw-milk bias."

By this time I suspect someone within FDA was asking this question:
"Who in hell decided to ask Mark McAfee to draft that press release?"

The regulators weren't through with their listeria campaign, except that
the next time it came up there was an even more amazing twist. In August
2008, New York's Department of Agriculture and Markets issued a press
release saying that, alas, *Listeria monocytogenes* had been found once again
in the raw milk produced by Lori and Darren McGrath. (It didn't allude to
the incident of the previous year.)[5]

Unbeknownst to Ag & Markets, Lori and Darren had instituted a policy
of retaining part of any milk sample taken by state inspectors, for just this
eventuality. (The milk they kept back is sometimes referred to as a "split
sample," since it's milk from the same sample taken by the regulators.) So
once the state's finding came back, the couple had the sample shipped to
a state-certified laboratory for the same test. Lo and behold, it came back
negative—no sign of *Listeria monocytogenes*.

I posted an account of what happened on my blog, together with a picture
of a hand caught in a cookie jar. I also quoted Gary Cox, a lawyer with the
Farm-to-Consumer Legal Defense Fund, who pointed out that it is very

difficult to use such discrepancies in court, since judges are reluctant to overrule regulators over something like test procedures, because there can be slight differences.[6]

Lori McGrath had the goods on Ag & Markets, but there wasn't much she could do with them. Her feeling was that Ag & Markets was simply sending a message to other dairy farmers who might be considering getting into the raw milk business:

> While I do not have any objection to any variety of testing, whether required by the State or requested by a customer, I do have considerable objection to inaccuracy of any degree. As most permitted raw milk farmers, we work arduously to maintain the utmost health of our herd, barn and milking parlor. If we cannot trust test results, how would we ever know if there was a true problem and/or how to resolve the issue?
>
> Interesting to me that most of our local friends and long-time farmers know exactly why we are being subjected to such annoyance. Needless to say, they won't be applying for raw milk permits.

Reading through these situations well after the events, I have to marvel that so much time and energy was being given over to a matter in which no one had even shown the slightest signs of illness. After so many incidents, though, I decided to try to find out more about *Listeria monocytogenes.* The studies I located suggest that, within the scientific and public health communities, the pathogen *L. monocytogenes* is viewed with much more skepticism than it is by state agricultural agencies like those in New York and California. Consider these concerns voiced in scientific papers and assessments:

A paper in the journal *Food Additives and Contaminants* reports that *Listeria monocytogenes* pathogens are "ubiquitous" in the environment and food processing plants and "foods are frequently contaminated." In other words, the little buggers are everywhere.[7]

So why don't we have frequent and massive outbreaks of listeriosis, the illness caused by *Listeria monocytogenes*? Well, not only do we not have frequent and massive outbreaks, we don't even have semi-regular or even occasional outbreaks. Listeriosis is quite rare, striking only five out of every *one million* people each year (or 0.00005 percent), according to the same study.

When it does strike, it primarily hits immuno-compromised individuals, as well as pregnant women and the elderly. And it hits with a vengeance, killing up to one-quarter of individuals who contract it.

Ironically, it's not known as primarily a raw milk problem. Quite the opposite. An outbreak of listeriosis struck Massachusetts consumers of *pasteurized* milk in late 2007, killing three. All three were elderly men. In addition, a pregnant woman lost her fetus. It seems the listeria had somehow multiplied in equipment being used to flavor the milk with strawberry and chocolate flavorings shortly after it was pasteurized.

The bottom line is that *Listeria monocytogenes* can contaminate pretty much any food. But if you are reasonably healthy, the chances of your contracting listeriosis are very slim indeed.

The reason there are so few outbreaks is that *Listeria monocytogenes* isn't an all-or-nothing problem. A few cells almost certainly won't make you sick. Here is how one scientific assessment published in the *Journal of Food Protection* put it:

> Because of the public health significance of *L. monocytogenes,* US regulatory agencies established a policy whereby ready-to-eat foods contaminated with the organism at a detectable level are deemed adulterated. This "zero tolerance" policy, however, makes no distinction between foods contaminated at high and low levels. . . . A microbial risk assessment based on the model shows that an alternative to the zero tolerance strategy has a greater risk reduction potential and suggests that a management strategy focusing on the concentration of *L. monocytogenes* rather than its presence alone may have a greater impact on the improvement of public health . . .[8]

In other words, don't waste time looking for a few cells in raw milk—rather, focus on spotting foods with high concentrations.

Even the US Food and Drug Administration, notwithstanding the stink it made about *Listeria monocytogenes* in the Organic Pastures cream, has expressed skepticism about the dangers from a few cells of the pathogen. In a 1992 commentary on a US Centers for Disease Control study about listeriosis cases in the nation, the FDA said,

> Whether a person becomes ill from *Listeria* depends greatly on an individual's health. Exposure to foods with *Listeria* does not automatically mean one will get ill. For most healthy people, a mod-

erate dose of *Listeria* bacteria on an ingested food is not likely to cause illness. The scientific community is still uncertain how many *Listeria* organisms it takes to cause illness; an infective dose varies with an individual's susceptibility. Exposure to high levels can make a healthy person ill, although such cases are extremely rare.[9]

Of the 1,850 illnesses and 425 deaths reported annually from listeriosis (as identified by the CDC study that the FDA was commenting on), most problems had originated with undercooked chicken, deli items, and "other ready-to-eat foods," along with assorted cheeses—presumably made from both raw and pasteurized milk.

Based on additional research, the FDA said nine years later in an analysis of "ready-to-eat foods" most likely to cause listeriosis that raw milk was "a moderate relative risk from direct consumption," and that fresh soft cheeses made from raw milk "have a higher degree of relative risk. . . ." Most producers of raw milk agree that soft cheeses, especially those imported from Mexico, are potential sources of pathogens that can cause disease, and they don't even try to produce them. Among other high-risk foods listed by the FDA were smoked fish, meat spreads, sausage, cooked ready-to-eat crustaceans, and vegetables.[10]

By late 2008, Chuck Phippen had experienced two additional positive findings of listeria in his milk, for a total of three instances over the two-year period. His fine was up to $500, except that he was refusing to pay, and was locked in a struggle with the New York Department of Agriculture and Markets. By early 2009, the Farm-to-Consumer Legal Defense Fund had taken up his case with the department. In correspondence with NYDA&M, Chuck used some of the same evidence from the scientific literature that I've cited here.[11] Then in May 2009, there was a fourth finding of listeria in his milk—with the milk sample being taken, amazingly, while he was at a meeting with top officials of the New York Department of Agriculture and Markets. As usual, no illnesses.[12] By the summer of 2009, Chuck told me he was up to six findings, and determined to continue fighting the state.

As I read these scientific assessments, and considered the fact that none of the customers of the raw milk farmers shut down by the state of New York in 2007 and 2008 became ill, I couldn't help but be suspicious of the treatment afforded Chuck Phippen, Dawn Sharts, Lori McGrath, and Mark McAfee. Especially since I have yet to hear about any other food producers being shut down for the simple presence of *Listeria monocytogenes* cells in their food products.

I wasn't alone in my concern. Ted Beals, a retired pathologist who had a long career as a professor at the University of Michigan and as National Director of Pathology and Laboratory Services at the US Department of Veterans Affairs, wrote on my blog after the August 2008 incident involving Lori and Darren McGrath:

> In ALL cases, by the time the regulators notify the dairy that they should stop distributing, all of the milk that was sampled has already been distributed. And additional tanks of milk distributed. And families (of all sorts) have already drunk the milk. And often all of the distributed milk has been consumed. And I am unaware of ANY examples of ANYONE becoming sick! And I tend to watch these cases. So here is the real disconnect. Dairies are being forced/ intimidated to stop distributing their milk because of a health risk, but there isn't any illness. This is what I am focusing on. Lots of possible explanations. Two I will suggest as starters:
>
> 1. The amount of pathogen in the milk is inadequate to cause illness (remember, most people who get raw milk don't just drink one glass we all drink lots);
> 2. The "pathogen" detected is present, but it isn't virulent. Lots of research showing that only SOME subtypes of the recognized pathogens account for the clinical cases.
>
> So where is the public health concern?[13]

Good question. Maybe the bigger question is this: Are we dealing with a public health issue or a political issue?

CHAPTER SIX

What Are We to Make of So Much Anecdotal Evidence?

In March 2007, I traveled to Michigan to meet some of the people involved in the Family Farms Co-op, including Richard Hebron, the target of the October 2006 sting operation.

The investigation of Hebron by the Cass County prosecutor, Victor Fitz, was still dragging on. As mentioned in chapter 4, Fitz had turned it into something of a national investigation, with inquiries to agriculture officials in Indiana, Pennsylvania, and possibly other states. To me, the longer it dragged on, the more dire the likely outcome. Prosecutors don't like to expend lots of resources investigating a case only to come up empty-handed.

Moreover, the previous month the US Food and Drug Administration had at long last responded to Senator Carl Levin's letter of complaint about the raid on Richard Hebron and the Family Farms Co-op, and its answer was one of defiance. "FDA, the Centers for Disease Control and Prevention, state public health agencies, as well as the American Medical Association and American Academy of Pediatrics, consider raw milk a public health safety hazard," it said. "In addition, FDA considers the cow-sharing agreements [which was the basis of the Family Farms Co-op] it has observed to be an attempt at circumvention" of a section of federal regulations that "prohibits the sale and distribution in interstate commerce of milk in final package form for direct human consumption unless it has been pasteurized."

In addition, the FDA had a few weeks earlier sent one of its "warning letters" to David Hochstetler, the Indiana raw dairy farmer who supplied the Family Farms Co-op. He was told to discontinue shipping milk via interstate commerce and, curiously, because of the advisory nature of what followed, was also told, "In addition . . . we have several comments concerning the lack of labeling of your raw milk and cream products." The paragraph then detailed alleged deficiencies by Hochstetler as to listing the name and place of his farm, net quantity, and ingredients on the milk container. It seemed as if the FDA was telling him not to ship his milk out of state, and to improve his labeling for milk distributed within Indiana.

Yet at a Friday-evening dinner I attended at the Ann Arbor home of one of my blog's early participants, holistic practitioner Linda Diane Feldt, the mood was fairly upbeat. Linda is a soft-spoken woman who has long been involved in a number of community activities, like teaching about food and health at a local high school and serving on the board of a different food co-op. She took community a step further by organizing regular Friday-evening community dinners, and about thirty or so members of the FFC attended this particular one.

Not surprisingly, there was lots of discussion about the fine points, and not-so-fine points, of raw milk consumption. One subject people had a lot of fun with was remembering the first time they had consumed raw milk. A few recalled with amazement their initial fears about drinking raw milk. "I thought I would get terribly sick," said one man. My own first experience was similar: I thought I might be poisoned by all the terrible bacteria lurking in this "illegal" drink. Then government regulators could claim, "See, we told you so." Not surprisingly, no one in the room had ever become even the least bit sick from raw milk, and many had been consuming it for a number of years.

Moreover, a number were doing what in public health circles is considered the unthinkable: They were raising their children on raw milk, and feeling good about it. More on this subject later.

Everyone seemed also to be in agreement that they could never go back to drinking pasteurized milk. One of the big topics of conversation, of course, was the legal case hanging over FFC, the threat posed by the prosecutor's investigation, and the FDA's hard line against the Amish dairyman David Hochstetler. FFC members feared these actions could lead to a disruption of their supply. "I've become dependent on raw milk," said one man. "My whole family has. I feel my children are healthier since they've been drinking it the last year or so. I know we couldn't drink the pasteurized stuff any more than we could drink Coke or Pepsi."

During dinner, Richard Hebron appeared, fresh from having dropped off milk for co-op members in Ann Arbor and Detroit. He looked to be in his early forties, but appeared younger than I expected, maybe because he had a thick salt-and-pepper head of hair and soft, almost radiant, skin for a man. It was an emotional experience to meet him—our phone conversations had created a bond. I admired his willingness to stand up to the authorities, and he was grateful to me for being pretty much the only media person keeping his case in the public eye.

Maybe it was because we were meeting in person, and he felt more comfortable talking, but Hebron confessed that the raid had hurt the FFC more than I had previously been led to believe, based on the public claims of support and solidarity by members. Immediately after the raid, demand for raw milk dropped by a quarter or so. Significant numbers of members opted out of the co-op, apparently afraid they might be caught up in the dragnet once state officials began combing through the co-op's business records, which they had confiscated during the search of Richard's home. These people didn't realize there's nothing illegal about *consuming* raw milk—it's the distribution that sometimes rests on uncertain legal ground.

In the intervening weeks, though, consumption gradually recovered. Richard told me that, based on that Friday's deliveries, consumption was down only about 10 percent from five months earlier.

Also attending the dinner at Linda Diane Feldt's was Steve Bemis, an FFC member who had been making comments on my blog. Bemis, a compact, slender man, was as serious and intense in person as he came across online. Raw milk had helped improve his health quite significantly, he said. "In early 2003, I began to have problems after every meal in the form of heart palpitations—butterflies in the stomach, or skipped beats." He tracked the problem to a gluten allergy and leaky gut syndrome, and so eliminated wheat and other grains from his diet to get rid of the palpitations. But he worried about the lost nutrition from eating fewer grains. "I tried raw milk and never looked back," he said. "In the first year of drinking it, my good cholesterol [HDL] went up from the low forties to the mid-fifties with no other change in diet. I'm also healthier, with very few colds, and when I get one, it's gone in a day." He couldn't understand why the government would be working so hard to deny raw milk to ordinary consumers.

In his "real life," Bemis was a pension lawyer with a large Michigan company (he has since retired), and he had been using his legal skills to advise Richard Hebron in his dealings with the county prosecutor, along with David Hochstetler in his dealings with the FDA. Indeed, Steve had just a few days earlier accompanied David to the FDA's Detroit office in an effort to convince the agency that milk being sent from David's farm in Indiana to Michigan wasn't for sale, but a regular distribution to cow-share members— and hopefully get the agency to change its stance.

Bemis also advised Richard Hebron to provide prosecutor Victor Fitz's office with testimonials from FFC members about why consuming raw milk was so important to them. He quickly learned a lesson that Mark McAfee, owner of Organic Pastures Dairy Co. in California, had learned several months earlier, when state public health and agriculture regulators shut his dairy down after six children who had reportedly consumed his milk became ill with *E. coli* O157:H7: Raw milk drinkers are very supportive of their special drink. Immediately after OPDC was cleared to resume sales in early October, Mark received dozens of letters from his customers, such as this from Pilar:

> It has been a wonderful day here, enjoying our pure, healthy, live milk! My oldest was especially grateful, as after four days of organic pasteurized milk he started acting autistic again and could not drink any more. The first thing we did when we got home from picking up our order from the buyer's club was open a beautiful carton of fresh whole milk and drink big glasses of it. I actually considered picking up a disposable camera and taking pictures of us enjoying the milk and sending them to you! (We don't have a digital.) Then I made a wonderful smoothie with the kefir and this afternoon we had popcorn with delicious raw butter all over it.
>
> For more testimony you can share with those learning about raw milk, I was fighting a cold last week, almost had it licked, and then I drank some pasteurized milk (dummy me). It was organic, but immediately I had the phlegm and the next day got laryngitis. I'm not kidding, as soon as I had some real live milk today, my voice started coming back. I don't know that I will ever buy milk again, unless it's raw.
>
> Thank you so much, and give the cows a big pat on the head from our family! (We refer to OPD as "Our" dairy . . .)

FFC members similarly weren't shy about responding. During late December and January, the testimonials poured in, some 232 in all.

You'd think reading through that many individual pleas to not prosecute Richard Hebron, and keep raw milk available, would be fairly tedious. But they turned out to be engrossing reading, with tales similar to what Pilar in California described—how raw milk had significantly improved all manner of seemingly intractable chronic conditions.

"Raw milk . . . literally saved my life," wrote Kathy. "I am a professional clarinetist with a national career—four years ago I was deathly ill with a chronic digestive disorder that threatened to end my career and my life. I had chronic pain for 25 years. I was able to rebuild my health to a vibrant state through the traditional foods from Family Farms Co-op and have been pain-free for three-and-a-half years."

An apparently elderly woman, Susan, wrote, "Since I've been consuming raw dairy, my health has improved dramatically. I have osteoporosis and am allergic to the medication the doctor prescribed. I feel so much better physically since I've been enjoying raw dairy. I no longer have muscle and joint pain . . . "

Jamie wrote, "I have been consuming raw dairy products for two years. I have noticed a significant decrease in seasonal allergies, asthma and inflammation since I have replaced commercially available pasteurized milk with raw milk and cream from pasture-fed cows."

Jill wrote: "I grew up a 'sick' child. Even though my parents thought that they were doing the best for me, the foods that I was being raised on were literally killing me. I was finally diagnosed as an adult with celiac disease and severe lactose intolerance. The pasteurized foods caused 25 years of distress in my gut (from the lack of lactase in commercial dairy) causing severe chronic abdominal pain, chronic fatigue, sleepiness, chronic tonsil infections, diarrhea, constipation—to name just a few. Since being on raw dairy, I no longer have these symptoms. My gut is getting healthier progressively, the more I feed my stomach these raw foods that are rich in enzymes. My sick gut is healthy now. If you take this blessing away from me, I'll be sick again. The pasteurization process destroys the enzymes my body needs to sustain itself. Raw dairy keeps me healthy so that I don't have to be a burden on society. Don't we already have enough sick citizens?"

Lou said, "Through raw dairy, I've experienced a dramatic increase in my health. In the summer of 2005, I was diagnosed with severe hypothyroidism. I used raw dairy as a way to regain my health. Almost a year later, I am almost off of all my prescription medications and haven't felt this good in years. As a matter of fact, I completed an ironman triathlon in October, using raw food for training food, with very good results."

The most curious to me were the letters from parents who claimed that raw milk made their children healthier. That was for me an ultra-sensitive area, I think because of the emotional upheaval surrounding the illnesses of six California children the previous September that public health officials linked to raw milk.

I recounted in chapter 2 the experiences of Mary McGonigle-Martin, mother of seven-year-old Chris. After Mary described his near-death experience, another California mother, Melissa Herzog, began commenting on my blog about how her ten-year-old daughter, Lauren, had had an experience similar to Chris, except her situation was colored by a modern-day American societal trend. Melissa was separated from her husband, and it seems Lauren had become ill while spending a September weekend with her dad and his girlfriend.

Melissa claimed Lauren became ill because the girlfriend had inadvertently served her raw milk that weekend (along with the rest of the girlfriend's family, who regularly consumed raw milk). More about this case in chapter 9.

But all I could think of after learning about this story was that a little girl might have become seriously ill when she drank unpasteurized milk for the first time. It fulfilled my worst fears. Those fears were fed further right around the time I visited Michigan when I had my own little encounter over giving raw milk to a child. I wrote this posting[1] about it.

What Do You Do When a Neighbor Wants Some of Your Raw Milk for Her Child?

I was catching up about a week ago with a neighbor I hadn't spoken with for a couple months because we had both been in winter hibernation mode. When I asked about her three-year-old son, she shook her head. "It's been one thing after another, sore throats and colds. We've been in and out of the doctor's office."

I inquired if she had ever thought of feeding him raw milk to build up his immune system, and she said no, but she was open to anything that might help. "I'll pick some up at Whole Foods," she said.

I explained that that wouldn't work, since we were in Massachusetts, not California, and then offered to get her some on my next trip to the New Hampshire farm where I obtain mine, in a few days. She seemed appreciative. (Interestingly, not many people I meet in the Boston area, including those who are otherwise very health-conscious, know much about raw milk and how limited its availability is.)

So I picked up my milk a couple days ago, but on my way back home, I got to thinking. What if the milk doesn't agree with her son or, worse yet, makes him ill . . . would I be responsible?

These events occurred around the same time that I published Mary McGonigle-Martin's recollection of how her son, Chris, had nearly died (see chapter 2). Here's what I concluded:

> It probably goes without saying that after reading Mary's terrible story, I decided not to give my neighbor any raw milk for her son. Instead, I decided to encourage her to buy it herself from a farm in the area.
>
> I take several messages from this ongoing, and passionate, discussion. For one, I think it's necessary to respect the power of what I might term "wild food" like raw milk. For whatever reasons, it can make people sick, especially children and others whose immune systems might not be fully operational. Just like wild-grown herbs and plants and fruit juice can make people ill. Of course, processed and cultivated foods (everything from tacos to spinach) can also make people terribly ill, and even kill them, though the causes are more likely manmade than nature-made.
>
> That leads to my second point, which is that these wild foods must be handled with care, especially when it comes to serving them to others who may or may not appreciate their power. As enthusiastic as I might be about the benefits of raw milk, I need to restrain myself in handing it out to others. I've taken to warning guests in my home who are interested in raw milk that they should try it first in small quantities; most are scared off by my cautionary words, since they were already nervous from a lifetime of pro-pasteurization propaganda. I feel badly, but then I realize they're probably better off making such decisions for themselves, not at my urging.
>
> All of which takes me to a third point, which is that the decision to consume such wild foods is likely best made as part of a larger decision about taking responsibility for one's health. And appreciating that with such responsibility comes risk.

A number of readers took issue with my characterization of raw milk as "wild food." Linda Diane Feldt, the holistic practitioner who hosted the dinner in Ann Arbor, wrote this comment:

> Cows eat lots of wild foods, but cows are the opposite of wild animals—they are so very domesticated. So I think your point about

raw milk being "out there" and a bit dicey to just share with anyone is right on. I just wouldn't call it wild.

I think of wild foods as actual wild foods—weeds and "seed themselves" plants growing in fields and woods, as well as game animals. Native and introduced plants gone wild. I make pesto from yellow dock, a version of spinach pie from dandelion, put plantain in salads, harvest stinging nettles in May with eager anticipation of this wonderful rich plant, dig burdock root for pickling and stir-frys, look for purslane as an omega 3 supplement, pick flowers of all sorts to add to salads. Wild garlic and garlic mustard will be up soon—yum.

I had to agree. My characterization of raw milk as a "wild food" was inaccurate. Maybe a better way to have expressed it would have been to say that it is a natural food that can be powerful in its benefits, but occasionally creates problems for children. Key to consuming it comfortably, though, is to be educated as to its many potential benefits and very occasional risks.

In the comments from the Michigan consumers in support of Richard Hebron, there were many parents who claimed their children were healthier after consuming raw milk. But clearly, these parents were highly motivated to seek help for their children via healthier food, and had made an effort to educate themselves.

"My son was considered to be lactose intolerant and had numerous ear infections when he drank pasteurized milk," wrote Kristin. "Since he has switched to raw milk, he no longer suffers from ear infections or any other illness. He doesn't seem to get sick like many children his age." Renee said, "My son is not able to drink pasteurized milk because the enzymes are destroyed in the pasteurization process and his body is not able to metabolize it. We have gone to the emergency room and he has been ill many times because of pasteurized milk. Pasteurized milk causes him to be unable to breathe, and he has had to be put on a nebulizer several times and use an inhaler many times. He also gets eczema from drinking pasteurized milk. Our doctor told us that these things were caused because he was allergic to milk. For years we avoided milk. After researching out healthy alternatives, we decided to try raw milk after reading of its benefits. He can drink raw milk without any of these problems. We have not been to the emergency room once from him drinking raw milk. My six children have not had one cavity since switching to raw milk."

Some accounts were very touching, like that from Michelle. "When my son's school therapists and some other family and friends suggested that my son was displaying symptoms of Asperger's syndrome and ADHD [attention deficit hyperactivity disorder], I began to research information on the Internet. I came across a study that maintained that [people with] Asperger's/ADHD are helped by consuming raw milk. I decided to purchase a cow share and try this with my son. Within two weeks, his therapists both asked me what changes we had made at home because he was a completely different person. He was more focused in his therapy sessions, he now made eye contact for the first time, and he was not flapping his arms while he walked. He was actually able to sit still. They continued to see improvement in him until the one month when I was unable to pick up my raw milk. He went without it for close to three weeks. Again, his therapists came to talk to me and mentioned that he was again very unfocused and more difficult to deal with. Once he was back on the milk, everything was fine again."

Some, like Lisa, spoke of seeming miracles in fighting serious disease: "I have an immediate, striking, personal reason [for supporting Richard Hebron]: In 2000 I was diagnosed with breast cancer. In August of 2006, the tumor was found in my bones. It looked widespread—pelvis, femur, scapula, spine, skull, humerus. But when the surgeon biopsied the sites, she found very few live cells, although they are there. Four biopsies later, there were still not enough live cells to get more specific information. What doctors have said is that my bones were keeping up with the destruction of the tumor cells. I don't take calcium supplements. The main source of bone-building material in my diet is the raw milk I've been drinking since 2003. A source of raw milk is essential for my health."

There was even a letter from a nine-year-old girl, Makenzie, in clear child's handwriting: "I think raw milk is 'the best.' We should be able to drink raw milk. My mom drank raw milk almost half her life. Raw milk is way more creamier than that organic [pasteurized] milk. They said on the back of that organic milk that it was creamy and smooth. That wasn't true at all. My cousin drank the store milk and got sick, but when he drank raw milk, he was just fine. We should have the right to drink raw milk."

Surprisingly, there were also letters of support from four medical personnel, two of whom were MDs, one a registered nurse, and one a naturopath. The medical establishment has been nearly unanimous in its opposition to raw milk. Yet one of the MDs observed: "In my 13 years of medical experience, I observed that pasteurized milk consumption has been linked to a host of illnesses such as chronic allergies, autoimmune diseases (rheumatoid arthritis, lupus), fatigue, thyroid problems, hormone imbalances, diabetes, arthritis, asthma, dermatitis, eczema and infections. When my patients switch to raw milk combined with comprehensive lifestyle and diet changes, symptoms often resolve or improve considerably."

The RN, Susan, provided both a personal and professional opinion: "Have you ever struggled to get a breath? Most people do not think about this, as breathing comes naturally, until you have asthma. I have adult onset asthma after being exposed to many patients smoking in the mental institutions and prisons where I worked as an RN for many years. This year, I had the wonderful fortune of being able to buy raw milk and grassfed meat. You cannot imagine the difference in my breathing. I can take a very deep breath without struggling. At my checkup this year, my doctor was very impressed with my improvement. 'What have you been doing to have such good oxygen saturation?' The only thing different is raw milk, true grassfed milk, and organic food."

A significant number of those who wrote in were simply outraged that what they saw as their fundamental rights were being abridged. Many expressed puzzlement and anger that the government would be interfering with their access to a natural food.

Julia started her mini essay with a question: "Has anyone been harmed by raw milk and organic meat? I'm wondering if the Michigan agriculture people can produce even one person who has been harmed by raw milk or the organic products offered by the Family Farms Cooperative. I challenge them to find someone. I used to work in a supermarket and I was surprised by the unhealthy choices most people made. The most frequently bought items in my store were Coca-Cola, white bread, and chips of all sorts. Whenever an order consisting mostly of fresh fruits and vegetables came down the conveyor belt, I would glance up and see who was buying them. More often than not, the people were speaking a foreign language or were clearly from another country. But in this country, we have the right to purchase cancer-causing, heart-attack-causing, diabetes-causing, obesity-causing foods, because we enjoy freedom of choice. There are vending machines laden with these unhealthy products in most American schools, and kids' lunch boxes are full of them. Governmental officials protect our rights to choose unhealthy foods because we are a free nation. Why won't they allow us to choose healthy, life-giving foods for ourselves and our families? I would ask them why they are harassing the farmers who provide these foods. Where is their evidence of harm?" Denise argued, "If the concern is for safety of consumers, we are the ones who have to be trusted to handle all of our raw foods safely. Just as when we purchase raw meat or vegetables. No one is going to come in my home and regulate what temperature I cook my meat to, or how I scrub my vegetables, or see what temperature I keep my refrigerator set at, or how old my leftovers are. It is up to me how I handle my food, whether it is raw or cooked. Now, I understand that there have to be some rules with the distribution of foods, and that's fine. I will follow any rules I have to, or sign any form I have to, but do not take away my rights to acquire food from farmers I respect and trust. If the issue is concern for my safety, don't worry, I've got it covered. If the issue is my rights, please do not take this communistic approach and try to control my purchase of food . . ."

As convincing and moving as these letters were, they were still statements on paper. More convincing are those from people you meet personally. I was fortunate to meet a number of individuals who say their families have benefited in ways large and small from consuming unpasteurized milk. One of the most moving meetings I had occurred during my March 2007 Michigan visit. In addition to meeting with bloggers, I was reporting on life at a small goat farm in Grand Blanc, about an hour west of Detroit, for a BusinessWeek.com series on family businesses. The owner of a lawn maintenance and snowplowing business, Rob Klaty, was working to convert an old horse farm into a raw goat's-milk dairy for members of a herd-share arrangement he set up.

When I walked into the small shed Klaty uses as a pickup spot for shareholders to obtain their milk, I encountered Brad Gill, a neatly appointed man in sweater and slacks. He was bent over a small white sink filling half-gallon glass jugs with milk from a stainless-steel vat above the sink.

Gill seemed standoffish at first, but gradually opened up about his difficult family situation. He was a Christian missionary worker, fifty-five years old, and lived in Livonia, a suburb of Detroit, about an hour away. He had a twenty-five-year-old son who was autistic and lived in a group home not far from Brad's home.

Gill said that he and his wife, Beth, didn't drink the goat's milk themselves, saving it all for their son. "Our son really requires this," he told me. "We are in a high medical need." Without the milk, he was prone to convulsions and bad behavior.

Much like special medicine, said Gill, the goat's milk "is a bit pricey, at $4 a half-gallon." And because of all the prohibitions, it's not conveniently available. To ease the driving burden, Gill alternated milk pickups with five other families facing similar medical issues.

"There's a bit of Americana here," Gill told me. "People getting together as a group, no one trying to beat anyone out or take charge or rule it. It's purely cooperative. There's a common need for the milk. We can't secure it as individuals," since raw milk of any kind, cow's or goat's milk, can't legally be sold in Michigan via retail outlets or even directly from farms. Only groups organized into herd shares can get at it, and when the herd-share supplier doesn't deliver to convenient drop-off points, like Richard Hebron of Family Farms Co-op, then carpools are essential.

There was still one category of raw milk consumers I wanted to meet: pregnant mothers who consumed pasteurized milk. I knew the Weston A. Price Foundation, a big proponent of raw milk, encouraged pregnant mothers to consume raw milk—on the order of a quart a day.[2]

Part of the reason I was so fascinated was that, in their warnings about the dangers about raw milk, the public health and medical establishments save their most dire warnings for pregnant women. In the FDA's list of people most at risk, pregnant women always come first, as in this warning: "The harmful bacteria can seriously affect the health of anyone who drinks raw milk, or eats foods made from raw milk. However, the bacteria in raw milk can be especially dangerous to **pregnant women** . . ." (The boldface emphasis is the agency's, with the list followed by "**children, the elderly, and people with weakened immune systems.**")[3]

I guess my desire to meet pregnant women who consumed raw milk was a little like my desire as a weekend skier to meet individuals who do so-called extreme skiing, where they are taken by helicopter to remote mountains with ungroomed trails and must find their way back to civilization. Like the extreme skiers, the pregnant women seemed to be on a crusade to test limits.

Yet when I met Valerie Walbek the following December in the parking lot of Oake Knoll Ayrshires Farm in Foxboro, Massachusetts—we were both there to pick up raw milk—and got to talking about how she had consumed raw milk during her pregnancy during most of 2007, she didn't seem like an extremist of any sort. Quite the opposite, in fact.

A slender blond woman of twenty-eight, Valerie explained that she had heard about raw milk a few years earlier from her mother-in-law, who gave her a tape of Sally Fallon Morell, the president of the Weston A. Price Foundation, speaking about common diet problems in our society. "I liked hearing about the history of raw milk and pasteurization and about the benefits of raw milk." Shortly afterward, Valerie and her husband, Daniel, had tracked down a farmer not terribly far from their home on Cape Cod who would supply them with raw milk.

Valerie and Daniel had mostly limited themselves to a vegetarian diet, so the shift to raw milk, along with Sally Fallon Morell's recommended grass-fed beef, was a big change. "I felt a lot better, I had a lot more energy," recalled Valerie about her new consumption of raw milk, raw butter, and grass-fed beef. "My skin was better, my hair was better, my menstrual cycle was more regular."

When Valerie became pregnant in late 2006, she had no hesitation about continuing with her habit of drinking two gallons weekly. "I'd be more concerned drinking milk from the supermarket," she says. "If I had the traditional American diet, I'd be worried about my baby . . . I felt I was doing the best I could for my baby."

What made Valerie especially fascinating is that she was a health care worker—a nurse practitioner in an office of obstetricians. So she was in the ironic position of advising other pregnant women about how to eat during pregnancy.

Like many raw milk drinkers, Valerie didn't broadcast that fact, and she stuck to that policy with her patients. "I counsel my patients to follow the FDA guidelines. I tell them to avoid raw milk."

She noted that her patients mostly have different outlooks than she has. Whereas she gave birth to her daughter Lucia at home, "The women I talk to mostly have planned hospital births. We all need to make decisions that make us feel the safest."

In fact, Valerie hadn't even told the obstetricians she worked for that she consumed raw milk. "I have mentioned I go to a farm for my milk, and not that it is raw. My goal is not to convert everyone. . . . I make decisions in my personal life that are different from what I tell women."

Based partly on Valerie's experience, I convinced the *Boston Globe Magazine* to publish an article I authored about the growing popularity of raw milk, especially for pregnant women. In the course of my research I learned via various raw milk consumers about a number of other women who had consumed raw milk during pregnancy.

One especially interesting person was Jennifer Klander, a thirty-year-old mother of two in the town of Chelsea, situated just a few miles north of Boston. What made Jennifer intriguing was that she was able to observe stark differences between her second pregnancy, when she drank raw milk, and her first, when she didn't. Her son, born first, in 2004, "was two-and-a-half weeks early, and he seemed kind of fragile and frail" at birth, she recalled. Her daughter was born three years later, at full term, and "was very strong and sturdy and robust, rosier and more solid" than her son.

The differences, she was convinced, were due to her raw milk consumption. So convinced was Jennifer, in fact, that she ignored pressure from her pediatrician to quit the raw milk habit. "My pediatrician is against us drinking raw milk at all," she told me. She and her husband steadfastly ignored the pediatrician's advice because both children were thriving from their own raw milk consumption. "My family has chosen to take the risk," Jennifer said.

The local evidence would seem to back her up. The Massachusetts Department of Agricultural Resources reports that the last known cases of illness from raw milk in the state occurred in 2001, when eleven Boy Scouts visiting a farm became sick from salmonella poisoning after drinking raw milk—all recovered. A more serious milk-related outbreak in Massachusetts occurred in late 2007, when listeria-tainted *pasteurized* milk killed three elderly people and caused a woman to lose her fetus.

The matter of risk is one that probably weighs most heavily on Terri Lawton, the farmer who produces and sells the raw milk that Valerie and Jennifer feed their families. Her family's farm, Oake Knoll Ayrshires Farm in Foxboro, Massachusetts—set amid ranch houses on a curvy tree-lined suburban street within two miles of Gillette Stadium, where the New England Patriots play football—dates from pre–Revolutionary War days, and is the last remaining dairy farm of any kind within Route 128, the highway that circles metropolitan Boston.

Terri is a husky blond woman in her late twenties who usually dresses in overalls and black rubber boots that come up nearly to her knees. She told me she gets special pleasure from watching pregnant women who have been consuming her dairy's raw milk since she began selling it in 2006. (Prior to that time, the dairy only produced conventional milk for pasteurization.) "One of the things I'm most proud of is that there are probably ten women who got pregnant while drinking our raw milk and gave birth to healthy babies who are growing fast."

Terri takes her responsibility—to produce safe milk—very seriously, as I observed beginning at five thirty on a wintry Friday evening in late December 2007, when I watched her milk her seven cows and bottle the milk.

The most important step, as in so many jobs, is the preparation. For Terri, the prep work took place in the unheated abandoned chicken coop that serves as the milk parlor. When I entered, I could see big puffs of steam rising from a large vat filled with plastic tubing and stainless-steel valves. I watched as Terri mixed in special cleansers with hot water and then washed, and rewashed, the milking equipment she was about to haul a hundred yards up an incline, to an old barn.

The tubing and valves would be used to automatically milk each cow and carry the milk first into a large glass container in a room adjoining the barn, and then the hundred yards downhill to a stainless-steel bulk tank in the milk parlor.

Terri wanted everything to be just right. "We try to do it the same every time," she explained. "If we do it the same today as we did it yesterday, then hopefully we'll get the same result."

The same result, of course, is clean, safe raw milk, but the challenge is scientifically immense. "We're trying to make sure something we can't see doesn't get into the milk."

Her customers are counting on her. Ask almost any raw milk drinkers why they would expose themselves, and their children, to the dangers and risks the FDA portrays—"like playing Russian roulette with your health," an FDA official has stated repeatedly—and they'll tell you it's because they have complete trust in dairy farmers like Terri Lawton.

"We did a lot of research" before deciding to make raw milk a family staple several years ago, explained Lyra Maclone, a thirty-three-year-old homemaker from Falmouth, who has a son, five, and a daughter, four. "We found a trusted source in Terri."

Lyra was reassured by the fact that the state conducts monthly tests of the milk that Terri and other raw milk dairies produce to measure bacterial levels. But this wasn't the deciding factor for her: "Even if they weren't testing, I would still be drinking it because I trust her. It's wonderful to be able to get that fresh milk, and [know] that it's coming from four or five cows, which is better than four or five hundred cows."

Yet as natural as the idea of young children drinking raw milk gradually came to seem to me, I was regularly reminded that it remains a totally repugnant idea to public health professionals. As one example, early in 2009, I wrote a posting on my blog[4] that referred to the growing acceptance of raw milk in the mainstream. As an illustration, I linked to a YouTube video[5] of young parents extolling the benefits of infant formula made from raw milk.

"Because of raw milk, we have a happy, healthy, and thriving baby," said the mother, Jenleen, standing together with her husband, Greg, and holding her son, Noah. The scene then shifted from their backyard near Los Angeles into her kitchen, where Mom demonstrated how she mixed raw milk together with other ingredients to create her formula.

The next day, I received an e-mail from a public health official who occasionally wrote when he thought I had strayed too far into pro-raw-milk territory: "When raw milk sites support raw milk formula, the regulators roll their eyes and push harder to ban the product/limit distribution (and conclude compromise is out of the question for 'those complete idiots')."

I had, not for the first time, touched the third rail of the raw milk issue—the matter of giving raw milk to young children, and, by extension, the matter of pregnant moms consuming raw milk. Even for public health experts inclined toward rational discussion, as this individual was, these are red lines. Their rationale: Adults can make the choice to accept the risks associated with consuming raw milk, but children and fetuses don't have that choice.

Such a knee-jerk reaction upsets devotees of raw milk, who feel they and their children benefit from its variety of good bacteria and enzymes. They see the parental decision to share raw milk with children as akin to similar ordinary but risk-laden decisions parents make for children, like driving them around in cars or giving them swimming lessons.

There is one other knee-jerk reaction common from the medical and public health communities, I discovered, when I occasionally provided examples of how individuals experienced health benefits from raw milk: the argument that these were "anecdotal" evidence, and thus not worthy of the same consideration as "scientific studies," which are based on large samples and/or include control groups against which to measure results. Indeed, in 2008 the American Academy of Pediatrics stated, in what can only be categorized as a diatribe against raw milk consumption, "there are no documented health benefits associated with ingestion of unpasteurized milk or milk products."[6]

Steve Bemis anticipated such reactions to his collection of consumer testimonials, presented to the Michigan prosecutor, when he summarized on my blog a tabulation he had done on the health benefits the cases communicated:

> I know it is not from a random sample (the respondents nearly all drink raw milk), nor placebo controlled or double-blind, but at some point the weight and number of "anecdotal" accounts rise above a mere story here and there. People do tend to have some

inkling of what is happening in their lives, and the lives of their children, whatever the scientists may think. There were a total of 232 testimonials submitted to Family Farms, both on the website and collected at the periodic cow-share deliveries, gathered in connection with defense of Richard's having been busted by the Michigan Department of Agriculture. We haven't done a sophisticated analysis of these results, but some initial tallying showed that fully half the respondents felt that their health, and the health of their families, was generally improved (fewer colds and flu, fewer ear infections, fewer doctor visits, fewer antibiotic prescriptions, etc.). More interesting, was that about 20% were able to drink raw milk in the face of previous lactose intolerance or other problems with drinking pasteurized milk. There was not one problem with raw milk consumption reported in these 232 testimonials . . .[7]

Dave Milano, a health care administrator and frequent commenter on my blog, pointed out in a comment in late 2008 that scientific studies haven't always driven scientific innovation:

In a somewhat playful letter published eight years ago in the British medical journal *The Lancet*, a physician made several comments regarding the value of anecdote that warmed my heart. He acknowledged that publication in a modern medical journal is "unlikely to follow anecdotal observation" but also made the point that a mere couple of generations ago, during a time when, not incidentally, many important medical discoveries were being made, it was very common to rely on anecdote as a base for decision making, and for inclusion in respected medical literature. Here is a quote from his letter:

"Observations can be criticized for being anecdotal. However, in the search for greater scientific objectivity, the habit of curiosity, once the very quintessence of medical discovery, may be lost."

The current inability (unwillingness?) of modern medicine to acknowledge the great and terrible "big picture" of [the] modern population's increasingly failing health indeed shows that the very quintessence of medical discovery has been lost. That vast empty hole has been filled with a dogmatic closed-mindedness, evidenced by blind trust in—even worship of—narrow, double-blind, controlled-variable studies. The trees have truly obliterated the forest.

Randomized studies can be valuable, but they are emphatically NOT all they are touted to be, especially when driven, as they undoubtedly are, by a near religious faith in early detection and medical management with drugs and surgeries as a solution for bad health . . .[8]

But it turns out there is, in fact, plenty of scientific research about both the benefits and dangers of raw milk. I'll examine that information in the next two chapters.

CHAPTER SEVEN

Is Raw Milk
Really Healthier?

Once I entered the world of raw milk, one of the first and most frequent claims I heard was that consumers of the stuff usually didn't suffer from lactose intolerance. I had never been lactose-intolerant myself, but I had heard enough advertisements for products like Lactaid to know it is a big problem for many people.

Sure enough, one of the major themes that stood out to Ann Arbor lawyer and co-op member Steve Bemis in the two-hundred-plus letters that Michigan consumers sent in to the Cass County prosecutor (described in the previous chapter) was how many of them referred to digestive issues associated with pasteurized milk—difficulties the consumers said were resolved with a switch to raw milk.

Bemis knew that lactose intolerance is a huge health issue—millions of people experience major intestinal discomfort when they drink pasteurized milk because they lack the enzyme necessary to metabolize lactose, a sugar found in milk. He also knew that the medical community's usual response to patients with lactose intolerance is to advise them to avoid dairy products, or else to seek out special pasteurized milk without lactose. Not a great solution if you love ice cream, whipped cream, and cream cheese.

Bemis determined that the sting operation against dairy farmer Richard Hebron, and the rising awareness of raw milk that resulted from it, afforded an opportunity to assess via a real-life study whether raw milk in fact alleviates lactose intolerance. With funding from the Weston A. Price Foundation, he teamed up with Ted Beals, a retired University of Michigan pathologist, during the summer of 2007 to launch a survey of members of Michigan and Illinois cow shares. The survey inquired into how many household members consumed raw milk, whether they had ever been told by a physician that they suffered from lactose intolerance, and, if they had, whether or not raw milk provided relief. Some 731 households completed surveys—they represented a total of 2,503 people—and, not surprisingly, 89 percent of those individuals were regularly consuming raw milk.

Bemis and Beals spent the fall and winter tabulating and compiling the results of this survey. Finally, by early 2008, they had some answers: Some 155 individuals, or 6 percent of the 2,217 regular consumers of raw milk, said they had been "told by a health care professional they had lactose intolerance." And, as the researchers suspected, raw milk had provided relief to many: Of the 155 with confirmed lactose intolerance, 127 exhibited no symptoms of lactose intolerance when they drank the fresh unprocessed milk. Yes, the sample size was small, but the results were clear. An overwhelming majority—some 82 percent—of those who had experienced feelings of bloating, nausea, gas, and other problems when consuming pasteurized milk had no such problems with raw milk.

Why was this a big deal? Lactose intolerance is a major food problem in the United States—some estimates are that as many as fifty million people suffer from it.[1] Because dairy is such a common item in our food—in cheeses, soups, cream sauces for meats and vegetables, cream for coffee, and an assortment of desserts, from ice cream to cakes and cookies—sufferers must be super-diligent about monitoring their diets, or risk encountering a bout of bloating and diarrhea just from eating cheese at a friend's house or a cream sauce in a restaurant.

To try to home in on just how big a problem lactose intolerance really is, Bemis and Beals engaged a national survey organization, Opinion Research Corp., to call a representative sampling of ordinary consumers. The organization determined that 15 percent of American households have at least one member who is lactose-intolerant. Based on that finding, Opinion Research concluded that about 10 percent of the US population, or about twenty-nine million Americans, have some degree of lactose intolerance (a somewhat smaller number than the fifty million estimated by the FDA, but still a significant number). Among children, Opinion Research extrapolated that the rates are even higher—some 18 percent of households with children, while the rate is 13 percent in households without children.

Lactose intolerance is just one of a number of chronic conditions afflicting many millions of Americans, especially children, and for a number of these conditions, rates of affliction have risen sharply in recent years. The mass media have been full of reports about alarming increases in asthma and allergies. For example, the Centers for Disease Control states that asthma rates in children have more than doubled since 1980, and that "the causes . . . remain unclear."[2]

Much of the rise in asthma cases is increasingly being attributed to the same factors that cause allergies: immune system problems. In many allergies, it's thought the immune response somehow goes haywire and mistakes peanuts or eggs for an infiltrating disease of some sort.[3]

A special report by *Newsweek* magazine about the alarming rise in allergies explained it this way:

> The cascade of events begins when an allergy-prone person encounters a substance like pollen or peanut. The body sees it as trouble and launches phase one of its offensive: the production of antibodies called IgE (immunoglobulin E). These molecules attach themselves to "mast" cells, which line the lungs, intestines, skin, mouth, nose and sinuses. The next time the person encounters the pollen or peanut, the mast cells are primed for warfare, sending out powerful chemicals, like histamine, which lead to those nasty allergic symptoms—wheezing, stomach cramps, itching, stuffiness, swelling and hives. . . . Fixing the immune system, so that it learns to distinguish good from bad without error 100 percent of the time, is every immunologist's dream.[4]

As the examples of the previous chapter suggested, many parents have embraced raw milk as a way to "fix" their children's and their own immune systems. No one knows for sure why raw milk seems to help individuals suffering from lactose intolerance. Unpasteurized milk contains harmless bacteria known as lactobacilli—which are killed off during pasteurization—and some research indicates that lactobacilli produce the lactase enzyme. This compensates for the insufficient lactase found in the digestive systems of lactose-intolerant persons, and helps these individuals break down and absorb lactose.[5]

Ron Schmid, in *The Untold Story of Milk,* says it's all pretty straightforward, based on his experience as a naturopathic physician: "Raw milk is rich in lactase, but the enzyme is destroyed by pasteurization. This is one reason raw milk is much easier to digest than pasteurized; in fact, most children and adults unable to digest pasteurized milk and diagnosed as lactose intolerant digest raw milk beautifully. This has been the case for hundreds of individuals I have worked with professionally."[6]

You'd think the tantalizing results Bemis and Beals had come up with might have become the basis for some further government- or university-sponsored research, to try to figure out exactly what was going on here. But that's not how things tend to work in the world of public health when raw milk is the issue.

Rather, the communication dynamic is something like what might have happened in the old Soviet Union, where you had to read between the lines and interpret hidden meanings in government publications. If you scanned the two main government papers, *Izvestia* and *Pravda*, you occasionally found a government reaction to some potentially controversial event that had occurred a month or two previously—maybe the arrest of dissidents or a crop failure.

In this same spirit, a month after I posted the results of the Michigan study on my blog,[7] in February 2008 the US Food and Drug Administration issued its version of a response.

It came in the form of a newsletter put out by the agency, *FDA Consumer Health Information*. Its main headline asked: "Problems Digesting Dairy Products?" Underneath, in somewhat smaller type, was the heading: "Does your stomach churn after you drink milk? Do you have diarrhea soon afterward? If so, you may be lactose intolerant."[8]

There followed two pages of background information about lactose intolerance—that an estimated thirty to fifty million Americans are lactose-intolerant; that it occurs because of an enzyme deficiency; and that it is most common in African Americans, Native Americans, and Asian Americans. It provided a list of common dairy products with lactose (ice cream, yogurt, milk, and cream.)

On the second page of the newsletter was the key item, a box with the heading: "Raw Milk and Lactose Intolerance." It started by quoting John Sheehan, director of the FDA's Division of Plant and Dairy Food Safety, as debunking claims by some raw milk advocates that pasteurized milk causes lactose intolerance. This is a viewpoint I hadn't heard from the raw milk community, but certainly it's possible that some advocates do blame pasteurization.

Written like a news article, it continued:

> Raw milk advocates also claim that raw milk prevents or cures the symptoms of lactose intolerance. Arguing that raw milk contains Bifidobacteria, they claim these microorganisms are benefi-

cial (probiotic) and create their own lactase, which helps people digest the milk. "This is not true either," says Sheehan. "Raw milk can contain Bifidobacteria, but when it does, the bacteria come from fecal matter (animal manure) and are not considered probiotic, but instead are regarded as contaminants." Drinking raw milk will still cause uncomfortable symptoms in people who are correctly diagnosed as being lactose intolerant. But worse than this discomfort are the dangers of raw milk, which can harbor a host of disease-causing germs, says Sheehan. "These microorganisms can cause very serious, and sometimes even fatal, disease conditions in humans."

What Sheehan seemed to be suggesting was that the individuals in the Michigan study who experienced relief from digestive problems likely weren't "correctly diagnosed" with lactose intolerance. In other words, there was no way raw milk could be providing relief from lactose intolerance. Those individuals experiencing digestive relief after consuming raw milk were presumably experiencing relief from some problem other than lactose intolerance. Or maybe they just imagined the problem, or the relief they were experiencing . . . or both. Adding insult to injury, as it were, according to Sheehan's analysis you could get so seriously ill from just consuming raw milk that it is "sometimes even fatal."

While there were legitimate criticisms that could have been made of the Michigan study, primarily the small sample size—155 lactose-intolerant individuals out of 2,217 raw milk drinkers suggests the study might best be used to point the way toward larger, more elaborate studies—Sheehan didn't seem to have those in mind. He was disdainful of any hint that lactose-intolerant individuals might have benefited from raw milk.

This little squabble about lactose intolerance was, unfortunately, just a tiny skirmish in an ongoing guerrilla war. The main battle is being played out most prominently in cyberspace, on the Web sites of the FDA and the Weston A. Price Foundation. It all started on the FDA's site, beginning in 2005, when the agency posted a sixty-nine-slide presentation—at once provocative and highly technical in its language—arguing that raw milk is no more nutritious than pasteurized milk, and is highly dangerous to boot.

Early on in its presentation, the FDA states: "Unfortunately, raw milk is sometimes marketed as being a 'health food,' and some raw milk vendors, when comparing their product to pasteurized milk, ascribe to it all sorts of curative properties, which are as yet largely unsubstantiated in the scientific literature."[9]

The heart of the FDA's presentation is thirteen "myths" about the comparative nutritional value of raw milk and pasteurized milk. "Myth No. 3," according to the FDA, is this: "Pasteurization inactivates enzymes that kill pathogens, including lactoferrin, xanthine oxidase, lactoperoxidase, lysozyme and nisin." In bold type, the FDA answers, "No, it doesn't" and cites a 1986 research paper to back up its contention.[10]

On its Web site, the Weston A. Price Foundation has countered with a seventy-one-page "response," in which it seeks to answer each of the FDA's arguments.

In commenting on the "health food" assertion, the foundation tries to explain the paucity of historical research: "Much of the research demonstrating the health benefits of raw milk was conducted prior to the 1960s and is therefore not indexed in databases such as *PubMed*. Modern experimental methods, tools of biochemical analysis, and methods of pasteurization are needed to reevaluate the question to the satisfaction of academic scientists and policy experts—but there is a large gulf between something that is 'as yet largely unsubstantiated' and something that has been refuted. The former implies that the claims have been partially substantiated and may be fully substantiated in the future."

The foundation also tries to emphasize a point I made in the previous chapter—that anecdotal evidence is worthy of consideration by consumers trying to sort through the sharply conflicting viewpoints and make a decision about whether they want to consume raw milk and feed it to their families.

"Many people who consume raw milk rely on anecdotal evidence of its superiority, including but not limited to their own experiences. Although anecdotal evidence is not sufficient to confirm a hypothesis, it is a valid means for generating one. Whether it is sufficient means for *acting* on one is a personal decision that every individual should have a right to make."[11] In other words, whether an individual decides to consume raw milk, or determines that the risks are too great, that decision ultimately should rest with the consumer rather than the government.

From that general face-off, the charges and assessments become ever more pointed. In its commentary on Myth No. 3 (how pasteurization kills off enzymes), the Weston A. Price Foundation points to two studies contradicting the FDA's contention—one it says "showed that homogenization only destroyed xanthine oxidase when it was preceded by heat treatment.

Pasteurization and homogenization of milk together destroyed 69% of the activity of this enzyme." Another study, from 2000, "showed that xanthine oxidase 'showed potent growth-inhibiting activity' against *E. coli* and *Salmonella enteritidis* at concentrations present in raw milk."[12]

"Myth No. 12" has it that "pasteurization makes insoluble the major part of the calcium contained in raw milk . . ." The FDA goes on to cite various studies indicating "there were no obvious differences in the absorption of nitrogen or the absorption and retention of calcium, phosphorus and sodium when compared to either raw milk or even a boiled milk . . ."[13]

The Weston A. Price Foundation wasn't about to be put off so easily. "Although this study did not demonstrate a statistically significant difference in mineral absorption, it did show that fat absorption was reduced by one-third when infants were fed pasteurized or boiled milk, which the authors attributed to the destruction of heat-sensitive lipase enzymes that are indigenous to raw milk."

The two presentations, not surprisingly, came to completely different conclusions.

The FDA concluded: "Many negatives are being assigned to the pasteurization of milk. Little, if any of it, is substantiable by the literature currently available."[14]

The Weston A. Price Foundation concluded, "While a few of the assertions may be unsubstantiated, the fact is that there exists an overwhelming set of observations recorded in the scientific literature justifying interest in the benefits of raw milk. There exist many anecdotal reports of potential benefits that the scientific establishment has not yet addressed. Consumers, however, should not be at the mercy of funding institutions that control which of these issues are researched; they should have the right to put into their bodies the milk of their choosing. Our federal and state governments, for their part, should be helping farmers produce raw milk safely, and the FDA should be providing us with a sober and balanced report on the safety and merits of raw milk rather than a piece of sensationalist propaganda."

Thus, the FDA didn't give credence to any of the evidence presented by the Weston A. Price Foundation. The Weston A. Price Foundation not only disagreed, but also pushed for giving greater credibility to anecdotal evidence. Clearly, this isn't just a scientific argument, but a political and consumer rights argument as well.

Because I tend to be holistically oriented—inclined toward disease prevention and natural healing via effective nutrition, and disinclined toward pharmaceutical approaches to disease, I want to believe that raw milk is nutritionally preferable to pasteurized milk because it's unprocessed.

I should add that I'm not obsessive about these beliefs. I've taken antibiotics when I've had bronchitis—something that used to happen every year or two. Since I've been drinking raw milk, beginning in 2006, I've had fewer of the coughs and colds that used to plague me, and those I've had have been milder than before, so I have avoided bronchitis entirely. But I would definitely still take antibiotics if necessary.

All this helps explain why I find the "story" surrounding raw milk so appealing. The idea that it is a highly nutritious product seems perfectly logical, since it is intended for calves, and is close in composition to mother's milk. Certainly there's little disagreement in most parts of the world that mother's milk is the best nutrient for infants, because it helps in key areas of development and also because it helps build infants' immune systems.

The other part of the story that makes sense is that raw milk, with its assortment of coliforms and other such "good" bacteria, serves as a kind of probiotic that helps maintain intestinal microflora. People all around the world have been aware for hundreds of years that natural probiotics like soured milk and buttermilk, along with fermented foods such as sauerkraut and other vegetables, are healthful—helping to strengthen immune system functioning and allowing for effective absorption of calcium and vitamins—because of the enzymes and the "good" bacteria they produce that populate your gut. The idea that the heat of pasteurization damages the bacteria and enzymes rings true as well.

The probiotic story was formalized during the last century. Dr. Elie Metchnikoff, whom I discussed in chapter 3 as having dissented from Pasteur during the 1880s about the germ theory, was very interested in probiotics. (Metchnikoff was awarded the 1908 Nobel Price in medicine along with Paul Ehrlich for their work in immunity.) In the early 1900s, he became intrigued with the fact that Bulgarian peasants who consumed lots of yogurt (made from raw milk, in those days) seemed to live long lives.

Metchnikoff developed a theory that aging is caused by toxic bacteria in the gut and that lactic acid could prolong life. He was so convinced of its veracity that he drank sour milk every day. He died in 1916 at age seventy-one, which was well above the average life expectancy of the general population at the time.[15] Another scientist from the Pasteur Institute, Henry Tissier, was the first to isolate a *Bifidobacterium*. He isolated the bacterium from a breast-fed infant and named it *Bacillus bifidus communis*.[16] This bacterium was later renamed *Bifidobacterium bifidum*. Tissier showed that bifidobacteria are predominant in the gut flora of breast-fed babies, and he recommended administration of bifidobacteria to infants suffering from diarrhea. The mechanism claimed was that bifidobacteria would displace the proteolytic bacteria that cause the disease.

Yet another scientist, L. F. Rettger, demonstrated in 1920 that Metchnikoff's "Bulgarian Bacillus," later called *Lactobacillus bulgaricus*, could not live in the human intestine, and the fermented food phenomenon petered out. Metchnikoff's theory was disputable (at this stage), and people doubted his theory of longevity.[17] As the germ theory took hold—with the ever-widening acceptance of pasteurization and the development of antibiotics through the 1930s and 1940s—the theory that all bacteria are dangerous took hold. The notion that there were "good bacteria" became ever less compelling.

Still, Metchnikoff's studies into the potential life-lengthening properties of lactic acid bacteria lived on in Japan, inspiring a scientist there, Minoru Shirota, to investigate the causal relationship between bacteria and good intestinal health. Convinced that a healthy balance of intestinal bacteria held the key to man's general well-being, Shirota dedicated his life and work to isolating a strain of lactic acid bacteria that would pass into the intestines, positively contributing to the balance of gut flora. In 1935, he succeeded in cultivating a unique bacterium, sufficiently robust to bypass the acidic environment of the stomach and enter the intestines directly. He placed this pioneering strain into a fermented milk drink in order to make its benefits accessible to all. This drink remains available worldwide today, in a recipe almost unchanged from Shirota's original formula, and is known as the Yakult drink.

An entire body of research has emerged on the benefits of probiotics in preventing illness. As one example, a 2001 study from the *British Medical Journal* of more than five hundred children enrolled in day care in Finland found that those fed pasteurized milk with probiotic added had modestly lower rates of respiratory and gastrointestinal infections than those fed milk without the probiotic. It concluded that adding probiotics to young children's diets "may reduce respiratory infections and their severity among children in day care."[18]

In another study, a group of researchers from Yale University and the University of Chicago published a paper in the journal *Nature* in 2008 showing that mice that had more of a certain friendly gut bacteria had significantly lower levels of Type 1 diabetes than mice lacking the bacteria. An executive summary concluded that "these findings indicate that interaction of the intestinal microbes with the innate immune system is a critical epigenetic factor modifying" predisposition to Type 1 diabetes.[19]

Perhaps most tellingly, in recent years large food companies have gone beyond touting the benefits of ordinary yogurt, which became very popular in the United States at the end of the twentieth century, and have begun pushing "functional" foods. The most prominent example is that of DanActive, a yogurt-like product that came on the market in the early 2000s.

"Helps strengthen your body's defenses," it says prominently on its package, adding in large lettering the term "Immunity." It then explains in smaller type: "About 70% of your immune system is in your digestive tract. This is where DanActive goes to work with the exclusive *L. casei* Immunitas cultures" (plus sugar, dextrose, and modified cornstarch).

According to the company's Web site, the notion that 70 percent of our immune system resides in our digestive tract is "a little known fact." As for the intriguing scientific name *L. casei* Immunitas, there's this explanation:

> There are many L. casei culture strains, some already present in human intestinal flora. First identified in 1919, L. casei strains are used in a number of dairy products worldwide. The L. casei Immunitas™ culture in DanActive is a proprietary strain that can only be found in Dannon's DanActive. L. casei Immunitas™ is the "fanciful" trademarked name for the L. casei culture that is only found in DanActive. . . . Multiple clinical studies have proven that DanActive with L. casei Immunitas™ can help strengthen your body's defenses."[20]

DanActive is owned by Groupe Danone, a European company with something on the order of $15-billion-plus in annual sales. Probiotics is a huge business in Europe. So if a $15 billion company is saying it's all about strengthening our gut flora, well, it must now be official.

As we saw in the testimonials I quoted from in the previous chapter, consumers of raw milk credit it with improving all kinds of conditions—allergies, asthma, colitis, autism, even cancer and heart disease.

The problem is that there has never been serious scientific research into most of these claims, like raw milk's effects on treating colitis, autism, and cancer. The recurring anecdotes and claims on behalf of raw milk even led at one point to a semi-humorous debate on my and another blog over whether raw milk might be useful in countering erectile dysfunction.

In a comment about President Barack Obama's likely view on raw milk, Mark McAfee, owner of Organic Pastures Dairy Co., wrote about the need for studies examining the role of hormones in conventional milk. Then he added this about raw milk:

> I know of many male consumers [who] have told me that our raw milk and or raw colostrum has been a [kind of] sexual Viagra . . . and that their male anatomy finally works after years at half mast . . . their wives also report that their level of health and sexual interest has been rejuvenated. Male or female . . . this is all about our human bodies working better and properly.
>
> I do not think that anyone studied raw milk and its estrogenic hormones as a whole food from cows on green grass pastures. I bet the studies were [performed] on pasteurized milk, which is a partial food that comes from the most unnatural sources.[21]

But leaving aside autism, cancer . . . and erectile dysfunction, in two areas, at least—asthma and allergies in children—there is an emerging body of important and scientifically recognized research on the impact of raw milk on health. It coincides with growing acceptance of the "hygiene hypothesis"—that children benefit from exposure to infectious agents and other microorganisms, and with little such exposure are more susceptible to developing allergic disease.

In the last decade, researchers documented an association between children from "farming environments" and protection against the development of allergies. The most recent, and impressive, in a series of studies was published in the academic medical journal *Clinical and Experimental Allergy* in 2007. It investigated "whether consumption of farm-produced products is associated with a lower prevalence of asthma and allergy when compared with shop-purchased products," examining results from nearly fifteen thousand children in five European countries. Among the farm-produced products was "farm milk," which is unpasteurized milk. (It should be noted that the researchers didn't clarify whether the unpasteurized milk was from grass-fed or grain-fed cows, nor did they determine whether some of the farm families might have boiled the milk prior to consumption.)

The results were conclusive, according to the study team of more than a dozen scientists from such prominent institutions as Harvard Medical

School; University of Basel, Switzerland; Zurich University Children's Hospital; and Karolinska Institute of Stockholm: "A significant inverse association with a doctor's diagnosed asthma was observed for all farm-produced products except vegetables and fruits. . . . When simultaneous adjustment was made for all farm-produced foods, only consumption of farm milk remained significantly and inversely associated with the prevalence of diagnosed asthma, diagnosed rhinoconjunctivitis, and current rhinoconjunctivitis symptoms."

Later in the study, the scientists again spoke of "evidence of a significant inverse association between farm milk consumption and childhood asthma, rhinoconjunctivitis, sensitization to pollen, a mix of food allergens, and horse dander. Other farm-produced foods were not independently related to asthma and allergy prevalence." Moreover, they said that "the inverse association was not explained by concurrent farm activities of the child or farm exposures during pregnancy and was most pronounced in children drinking farm milk since their first year of life." In other words, it wasn't just the cleaner air or dirtier dirt of farms, it was the milk.

What was it about the milk? They said they couldn't be sure. "At present, we can only speculate about the components of farm milk responsible for the observed protective effect. Farm milk possibly contains different levels or a different composition of pathogenic and nonpathogenic microbes compared with milk purchased in a shop."

The scientists followed this theme through in their closing remarks: "In conclusion, the results of the present study indicate that consumption of farm milk is associated with a lower risk of childhood asthma and rhinoconjunctivitis. These results might be transferred to non-farming populations . . ."[22]

These results so impressed a scientist at the University of London who had carried out his own research in 2006 to try to isolate the areas of the farming lifestyle to explain the reduced incidence of childhood allergies, he wrote an editorial in a 2007 issue of *Clinical and Experimental Allergy*, "Unpasteurized Milk: Health or Hazard?"[23]

The scientist, M. R. Perkin, acknowledged "the allergy epidemic" in the United States and United Kingdom in pointing to "the small but growing body of evidence that consumption of unpasteurized milk is another factor mediating a protective effect on allergic disorders."

He raised two nearly heretical issues: "What is it about unpasteurized milk consumption that confers a protective effect, and why is the effect heterogeneous depending on the country and population studied?" The latter question was asking, in effect, why raw milk seems to work on children, regardless of where they live or their race or ethnic background.

Perkin pointed to evidence that raw milk differs significantly from pasteurized milk in terms of its nutritional composition. "Grass-fed cattle produced milk with a higher ω-3 fatty acids content," which "reduce prostaglandin formation by competitive inhibition with ω-6 fatty acids (linoleic acid) and by inhibiting the action of cyclo-oxygenase." In addition, "unpasteurized milk differs from pasteurized milk in its content of a number of other substances. Paradoxically, in addition to containing a higher microbial load, unpasteurized milk contains antimicrobial substances (lactoferrin, conglutinin, lactoperoxidase and free short-chain volatile fatty acids)." (As I noted earlier, it's not known whether the cows in the European study on allergies were entirely grass-fed.)

While some raw milk advocates actually blame pasteurized milk for triggering the epidemic of allergies and other chronic conditions, Perkin takes issue with them, noting, "The adoption of pasteurization in the milk industry would seem to predate the onset of the allergy epidemic by too significant a period of time for it to be causally related to the epidemic."

But the same can't be said for homogenization, which came into widespread use in the 1940s and later. "A closer temporal relationship could be argued for the homogenization process," he says, and goes on to consider the chemical and structural changes induced by homogenization, which "causes a reduction of fat globule size and a concurrent increase in the milk fat surface area, which alters the original milk fat globule membrane . . ." The bottom line is that "the homogenization process could be inducing changes in cows' milk that might have a deleterious immunological effect."

While such comments from established scientists and established scientific journals stand out sharply in this day and age, with the scientific establishment nearly entirely hostile to raw milk, it needs to be noted that they contain an important "however."

This "however" stems from the logical question that arises from the research: If raw milk helps reduce childhood asthma and allergies (which together affect an estimated sixty million Americans),[24] why not recommend it as a way to reduce those risks? Certainly it would seem preferable to the powerful drugs children take to alleviate these conditions.

And the reason, say the scientists who carried out the European farm study in their conclusion, is that "raw milk may contain pathogens such as salmonella or [*E. coli* O157:H7], and its consumption may therefore imply serious health risks."

They didn't slam the door completely shut, though, allowing that "A deepened understanding of the relevant 'protective' components of raw milk and a better insight into the biological mechanisms underlying the reported epidemiological observation are warranted as a basis for the development of a safe product for prevention."

M. R. Perkin in his editorial was even more adamant in encouraging further assessment of raw milk's preventive powers:

> Yet a paradox remains. Clearly, a dairy farming family's propensity is to ignore governmental advice and utilize this essentially free resource. This paper adds to the weight of evidence that a protective effect is associated with unpasteurized milk consumption. The potential of identifying the underlying mechanism that yields a two-thirds reduction in sensitization must be worth pursuing. The key issue now is to determine what underlies this protective effect and whether it is possible to separate the protective from the potentially hazardous elements.[25]

As I said, it's difficult to overstate the importance of such research findings and the favorable statements of well-regarded scientists. Whether it was because of these articles or the rapidly growing interest in raw milk, America's medical and scientific establishments came out in 2008 with a literal barrage of adamant objections. First, Harvard Medical School published an article on the widely read Microsoft Network via its Harvard Health Publications, which supposedly answered a question by a parent about serving raw milk to children. It concluded: "There are parents who believe raw milk is more nutritious than pasteurized milk. Research has shown this is not true. There is no nutritional advantage to drinking raw rather than pasteurized milk."[26]

Not long afterward, in December 2008, the American Academy of Pediatrics published an article in its "official news magazine" telling its members in a heading, "Advise families against giving children unpasteurized milk."[27]

It used language similar to Harvard Medical School in concluding that "there are no documented health benefits associated with ingestion of unpasteurized milk or milk products."

Then, in January 2009, the scientific journal *Clinical Infectious Diseases* published an article titled "Unpasteurized Milk: A Continued Public Health

Threat" in which it concluded: "Scientific evidence to substantiate the assertions of the health benefits of unpasteurized milk is generally lacking."[28]

What is interesting about this particular paper is that it at least acknowledges the growing popularity of raw milk: "Despite the overwhelming scientific understanding of pathogens in milk and the public health benefits of pasteurization, there is considerable disagreement between the medical community and raw-milk advocates concerning the alleged benefits of consumption of raw milk and the purported disadvantages of pasteurization."

But interestingly, none of the bastions of establishment health and science confront the very real research showing the benefits of raw milk. The closest thing to an objective assessment of the research has come from an attorney prominent in the food-borne illness world, Bill Marler of Seattle firm MarlerClark. The firm has represented families who became ill from raw milk. He runs several blogs on food-borne illness, and on one of them, he published a review of research assessing the benefits of raw milk. Given his anti-raw-milk orientation, he had some favorable things to say.

"There is substantial epidemiological evidence from studies in Europe that consumption of raw milk products in childhood has a 'protective' effect for some allergic conditions (e.g., asthma, hay fever, eczema)," he said in the 2008 assessment. He added, "Raw milk and cheeses may contain microflora ('beneficial bacteria') that produce metabolites and other antibacterial compounds that may be toxic to food-borne pathogens."[29]

American establishment scientists could argue, for example, that the research isn't complete enough, or has flaws. But they don't do that. Instead they repeat the contention that no research exists to support the possibility that raw milk confers health benefits, when clearly that is a lie.

All of which raises this question: If you can't believe what they say about the existence of research supporting the nutritional benefits of raw milk, can you believe what they say about the dangers of raw milk? That is the subject of the next chapter.

CHAPTER EIGHT

How Dangerous Is Raw Milk, Really?

As the renewed state and federal government campaigns against raw milk unfolded in 2006, Pete Kennedy was becoming ever more upset. Kennedy worked as a lawyer retained by the Weston A. Price Foundation to help raw dairy farmers deal with the legal problems posed by regulator crackdowns, and he was getting an increasing number of calls from dairy farmers whose operations had either been shut down or were threatened with shutdown by the government's aggressive strategies, as described in chapter 1: lab reports of listeria contamination, without any evidence of consumer illnesses; or regulator claims of illegally selling raw milk products like yogurt and butter. (By early 2008, Kennedy had become the director of the Farm-to-Consumer Legal Defense Fund, an organization formed July 4, 2007, in part with support from the Weston A. Price Foundation, to seek legal redress for owners of small farms against government threats.)[1]

I first came into contact with Kennedy in fall 2006, following the tough enforcement actions against raw dairy farmers in California, Michigan, and Ohio. A bookish-appearing guy with tousled brown hair, he told me he had just in the last few years transitioned to using his legal training after years running a small business. During the previous summer of 2006, what was most bothering Kennedy was the increased shrillness and frequency of the federal and state warnings about raw milk. "They keep saying how much more dangerous raw milk is than pasteurized milk," he explained to me in one 2006 conversation we had about a raw dairy farmer's problems.

Never, though, did the government warnings say anything about the dangers of pasteurized milk, he noted. Pasteurized milk? I wondered. Why should we be concerned about pasteurized milk? After all, isn't the entire purpose of pasteurization to kill all the germs that could create problems?

It turns out there have been a number of well-documented cases of serious and widespread illness from pasteurized milk, and Kennedy rattled off several for me.

For instance, in 1983, fourteen of forty-nine Massachusetts residents who had contracted listeriosis from pasteurized milk died. The *New England Journal of Medicine*, in a 1985 writeup of the case, expressed open concern about the fallibilities of pasteurization: "The milk associated with disease came from a group of farms on which listeriosis in dairy cows was known to have occurred at the time of the outbreak," said the article. "Multiple sero- types of *L. monocytogenes* were isolated from raw milk obtained from these farms after the outbreak. At the plant where the milk was processed, inspec- tions revealed no evidence of improper pasteurization. . . . These results support the hypothesis that human listeriosis can be a foodborne disease and raise questions about the ability of pasteurization to eradicate a large inoculum of *L. monocytogenes* from contaminated raw milk."[2]

And then there was a case two years later in Illinois, which, according to the *Journal of the American Medical Association*, led to sixteen thousand confirmed illnesses of salmonella infection—traced to 2 percent milk from a single dairy. In fact, the toll was likely ten times that, reported the JAMA authors. "Two surveys to determine the number of persons who were actu- ally affected yielded estimates of 168,791 and 197,581 persons, making this the largest outbreak of salmonellosis ever identified in the United States," the article summarized. Further investigation showed that the same strain of salmonella had contaminated the plant for at least ten months "and repeat- edly contaminated milk after pasteurization."[3]

There was an even worse case in 1994 described in the *New England Journal of Medicine*—one in which 224,000 people around the country became ill from salmonella contained in Schwan's ice cream. After much testing of the ice cream samples, the ice cream plant, and the tanker trailer trucks that transported the ice cream premix, the investigators couldn't be sure which part of the dairy concoction was at fault, though they leaned toward the egg component. "This nationwide outbreak of salmonellosis was most likely the result of contamination of pasteurized ice cream premix during transport in tanker trailers that had previously carried nonpasteurized liquid eggs containing *S. enteritidis*."[4]

There have been other equally shocking cases of illness in which pasteur- ized milk was a major factor in triggering illness. In May 2006, more than thirteen hundred prisoners in eleven California facilities around the state became ill with campylobacter (sometimes referred to as a *C. jejuni* infection).

A preliminary report by California scientists, presented as an abstract at a meeting of the American Society for Microbiology in 2007, said the infection was traced to "post-pasteurization contamination of the milk" produced by the prison system's own dairy, possibly from inappropriate manure management practices. As in so many other such cases, the actual source hasn't been traced. An Associated Press story speculated that the milk was spoiled.[5]

While all the sickened inmates in California recovered, that wasn't the case in a 2007 Massachusetts outbreak of illness from pasteurized milk. As I've noted previously, over the course of about six months three elderly individuals died and a young mother-to-be lost her child in a miscarriage from the listeriosis they contracted from drinking pasteurized milk. Investigators eventually traced the listeria pathogen to flavorings added to the milk after pasteurization.

Kennedy was also bothered by the fact that the FDA's PowerPoint presentation on raw milk, which I discussed at some length in the previous chapter in relation to the health benefits of raw milk, makes no mention of any of these cases, or even that people can and do become ill from pasteurized milk. While the FDA presentation is titled "On the Safety of Raw Milk (With a Word About Pasteurization)," its entire purpose seems to be to cast doubt on raw milk.[6] It concludes with the provocative statement made famous by John Sheehan, the FDA's plant and dairy manager: "Drinking raw milk or eating raw milk products is like playing Russian roulette with your health."[7]

Kennedy noted that the FDA presentation goes through study after study and outbreak after outbreak indicating that raw milk is dangerous, even though the evidence from a number of the studies appears tenuous at best, according to the Weston A. Price Foundation's point-by-point response.[8]

For example, several salmonella outbreaks referred to in the FDA presentation involved Mexican-style fresh cheeses (*queso fresco*) made from raw milk—sometimes referred to as "bathtub cheese." These cheeses are popular among Hispanics, but often they are produced under unsanitary conditions. "There are many opportunities for cheese to be contaminated even if the milk is pasteurized—especially if the cheese is made in a home kitchen," says the Weston A. Price Foundation's response. Serious producers of raw milk—the kind of dairy farmers who were being hit on by the government regulators—generally disassociate themselves from such cheeses because of the farmers' focus on maintaining the highest possible sanitation levels.

In addition, a number of raw milk outbreaks cited by the FDA may have resulted from individuals consuming milk not produced by the special dairies Kennedy was familiar with, but rather by conventional dairies where sanitary practices were questionable because their milk was intended for pasteurization's "cleanup." The FDA slide show reported on a 1982 study indicating that when certain bacterial infections in the United States between 1979 and 1980 were examined, "They indicated that when exposure to cattle, beef or dairy products was examined, cases differed significantly from controls only by a more frequent consumption of raw milk."[9]

The Weston A. Price Foundation's response to that study's interpretation noted, "Eight out of twelve subjects who drank raw milk obtained it from 'a local farm that was not intended for commercial sale.' The authors made no investigation of the sanitation or feeding methods at these farms."[10]

The reason this point is so important is that there are really two categories of raw milk in the United States. One is conventional milk intended for pasteurization; the second, raw milk intended to be sold unpasteurized. Dairy industry studies have shown that raw milk of the first kind, which is really almost all milk produced in the US, has significant rates of pathogen contamination before pasteurization. A study published in a 2004 issue of the *Journal of Dairy Science* found that in milk samples taken from 861 bulk tanks in twenty-one states around the country, 2.6 percent contained salmonella and 6.5 percent tested positive for *Listeria monotcytogenes.* While the presence of pathogens "was low," according to the study's authors, it is important to keep in mind that the dairies sampled produce their milk with the expectation it will be pasteurized. Thus, while the *Journal of Dairy Science* noted that the contamination "highlights the need for vigilance in maintaining hygienic conditions in milking and processing environments," the reality is that the farmers whose milk contained the pathogens could rest assured that the milk wasn't a public health hazard because it would be pasteurized. Thus, the incentives for developing excellent sanitation were less than they are for farmers intending their milk to be sold raw.[11]

The FDA presentation actually highlights on one of its slides the dangers associated with diverting raw milk destined for pasteurization for use in making "bathtub cheese."[12]

According to the Weston A. Price Foundation's response, this dangerous situation takes place because makers of the soft cheese often acquire milk from providers whose milk is intended for pasteurization. The cheesemakers

> use the false claim that they need milk to feed to young livestock in order to convince large dairies to sell them unpasteurized milk under

the table. They load up the purchased milk into pickup trucks full of plastic 19-liter buckets. A farm that produces 20,000 to 40,000 liters of milk per day may sell about 200 liters to unlicensed cheesemakers this way. The farmer earns $12 per bucket, which is double the price he gets for selling the milk to a processing plant. Raw milk illegally taken from a source that is intended for pasteurization *is* unsafe. The open and legal sale of raw milk produced according to high standards is the safest solution to the public demand for nature's perfect food.[13]

Kennedy criticized the tendency of the government to categorize illnesses as coming from raw milk when the evidence often wasn't so clear. For example, on one slide describing a study of 1,333 Wisconsin residents who had contracted *E. coli* O157:H7, it concluded, "Among case patient identifiable exposures, consumption of raw milk/milk products was among the top three causes most frequently noted, at 7% of cases."[14]

To which the Weston A. Price Foundation responded, "This study did not identify the causes of any of the 1,333 infections. The authors simply compiled the cases that were reported during this time period. They identified risk factor information in addition to that which was originally reported by reviewing case follow-up forms. They did not provide any information about the content of these forms except that they ascertained whether the patients had drunk unpasteurized milk or had contact with other infected patients in a daycare setting."[15]

Kennedy noted that, in addition to the various failings of the FDA presentation, nowhere in it is there any kind of statistical analysis of where raw milk fits in terms of the overall dangers posed by food-borne illnesses. In other words, how does raw milk rank in danger compared not only with pasteurized milk, but also with chicken, hamburger, salami, sushi, and so forth?

As government regulators focused ever more harshly on raw milk producers, Kennedy decided it could be useful to compare the number of illnesses from raw milk versus pasteurized milk. But there seemed to be little hard data available on actual disease incidence from either raw milk or pasteurized milk. Indeed, there's almost no data even on the number of raw milk drinkers in the United States. There have been some efforts to extrapolate numbers, as you'll see later in this chapter, but they are far from precise.

The most recent study on disease outbreaks from raw milk appeared to have been a 1998 review from the *American Journal of Public Health*. The study analyzed raw milk outbreaks reported to the CDC between 1973 and 1992. It reported data from twenty-one states, with the total number of illnesses over the twenty-year period being 1,733, or an average of about 87 per year. Raw milk consumption was estimated to be less than 1 percent that of pasteurized milk.[16]

Kennedy not only wanted these figures updated, but he also wanted to see how raw and pasteurized milk fit into the big picture. So in July 2006, he decided to obtain real data comparing the incidence of illness from both raw milk and pasteurized milk. The best approach, he determined, was to put in a Freedom of Information Act (FOIA) request to the federal Centers for Disease Control in Atlanta. Any citizen can make an FOIA request. He asked for a tally on the number of food-borne outbreaks associated with pasteurized and unpasteurized milk between 1973 and 2005—a total of thirty-three years.

Months went by, with no response. Finally, in May 2007, ten months after his request, Kennedy received a mailed response: five pages of tables showing, year by year, the number of food-borne outbreaks from pasteurized and unpasteurized milk "reported to the CDC's National Foodborne Outbreak Surveillance System, 1973–2005."

After spending several weeks digesting the information, Kennedy alerted me in July that he was ready to release it publicly. To me, the report was stunning in a key revelation: Raw milk's contribution to the nation's foodborne illness problem was minuscule.

The central question that Kennedy analyzed was this: How many Americans become ill in an average year from raw milk contamination, whether it be from *E. coli* O157:H7 or campylobacter or salmonella or listeria? We're not talking about deaths here, we're talking illnesses.

The answer is: fifty-four persons. And if you take out the average of five per year who became sick from eating imported Mexican cheese, that number shrinks to forty-nine.

Those are the numbers that come out when you average official government statistics showing 1,791 total illnesses from raw dairy and 1,609 raw milk illnesses over the thirty-three-year period between 1973 and 2005.

In fact even these figures may be high, since the government in its cover letter hedges, saying, "Food vehicles identified are not necessarily confirmed with statistical or epidemiological evidence."

As for pasteurized milk, there are something on the order of six hundred illnesses on average per year, more than ten times the average for raw milk (though surely not as high on a per capita basis as raw milk illnesses).

Kennedy points out that the number of illnesses from raw milk and pasteurized milk "is still minuscule compared to the overall numbers" of people made ill in an average year by food-borne illness, which the CDC estimates at seventy-six million. "Some hundreds of thousands of people are consuming raw milk," Kennedy says. "It seems like the government's campaign against raw milk is an overreaction and is motivated by something other than science and health." What else could possibly be motivating the government?

As always in the debate over raw milk, the numbers were assessed for better, or worse, depending upon whom I consulted. Pete Kennedy was convinced that even the 1,609 total illnesses was likely a high number. "These are based on reports from state public health officials," he told me. "In many of those cases, public health [officials] surmise that raw milk is the cause of illness. You saw the cases in Ohio, for example, the boy who was eating snow [possibly contaminated] with bird feces [see chapter 2]. The officials decide that's from raw milk because he happened to also drink raw milk. So their numbers are often inflated."

On the other side of the fence, epidemiologists argue that reported cases are only the tip of a very large iceberg. Michele Jay-Russell, a food safety and security researcher with the Western Institute for Food Safety and Security at the University of California–Davis, argues that the average of forty-nine annual illnesses from raw milk almost certainly understates the actual situation, and that comparing that number with the total estimated seventy-six million illnesses from food-borne illness is

> comparing apples and oranges. Lots of people make this mistake because it is confusing. The 76 million number comes from projections/estimates based on many factors. The 49 number comes from actual reported cases listed in CDC's database. But because so many cases go unreported, researchers build in a "multiplier" for the likely real number of cases. For example, one research approach has the multiplier for *E. coli* O157:H7 underreporting as 20. So if there were 205 illnesses reported in the spinach outbreak, the estimated number would be 4,000 illnesses of those 76 million per year. The multiplier for salmonella is higher—40 times.

Actually, the numbers Kennedy obtained are somewhat lower on an average annual basis than those published in the *Journal of Public Health*

I quoted earlier in this chapter. That paper reported 1,733 illnesses from twenty-one states over a twenty-year period from 1973 to 1992, while the CDC numbers Kennedy obtained reported 1,791 nationwide over thirty-three years. Since Kennedy obtained the CDC data, additional data has come out; the numbers seem to be in a similar range.

At a symposium on raw milk sponsored by the International Association for Food Protection in February 2009 (with the reassuring title: "Raw Milk Consumption: An Emerging Public Health Threat?"), Caroline Smith DeWaal, food safety director of the Center for Science in the Public Interest, reported that between 1990 and 2006 there were 1,570 illnesses from unpasteurized dairy products tabulated by her organization. At least another forty-five hundred illnesses were caused by pasteurized dairy, she said. Once again, the numbers are in the same general range as those reported by the *Journal of Public Health* and the CDC data.[17]

Like Michele Jay-Russell, Smith DeWaal pointed out that "a minority of outbreaks make it into the CDC database." She cited additional concerns as well: "Dairy outbreaks increased dramatically in 2005 and 2006, in large part due to a rise in outbreaks from unpasteurized dairy products." In addition, "Dairy products identified as unpasteurized were associated with 30% of the dairy outbreaks, including nearly 70% of milk outbreaks."

Smith DeWaal argued, as did another presenter, that many more illnesses from raw milk occur in the roughly half of states (the actual number is continually changing) that permit sales of unpasteurized milk either directly from the farm or via retail channels. "Nearly twice as many [illnesses] occurred in states that allow raw milk sales," she stated.

The matter of where raw milk illnesses are likeliest to occur was the subject of another presenter at the same symposium, CDC scientist Adam Langer. He provided an analysis asking, "Do State Raw Milk Sales Restrictions Reduce Raw Milk Outbreaks?" He went through a complicated statistical analysis—"incident density ratios" and other such mathematical devices—to finally conclude that if you live in a state that allows raw milk sales, the risk of getting sick from raw milk is on the order of two to three times greater than if you live in a state that prohibits such sales.

To my way of thinking, if you live in a state that prohibits the sale of hamburger meat, you'll have a lower incidence of illnesses from hamburgers than you'd have in a state that allows sale of hamburger meat. Indeed, you could apply that principle to any food you can think of that might occasionally make you sick. However, Langer's dire prediction was crystal-clear:

If raw milk sales were to be extended to states that now prohibit the sale, "There would be an increased risk threat throughout the country."[18]

In the end, Smith DeWaal of the Center for Science in the Public Interest countered her own concerns by pointing out that, in the whole scheme of food-borne illness, dairy products overall play a small role. In fact, dairy products, both pasteurized and unpasteurized, account for only about 4 percent of all food-borne illnesses in the United States. "Produce is four times more likely and seafood thirty times more likely to get you sick than dairy," she said.

One reader of my blog, Greg Bravo, took Smith DeWaal's assessment a step farther in comparing the dangers of raw milk to other foods. He used some CDC data to begin calculating the dangers presented by raw milk versus other foods, along with the number of raw milk drinkers in the United States.[19] Using a presentation by a professor at Colorado State University, he guided readers to information contained in a summary table.[20]

> This table gives total cases of listeria in the US, as well as their food source. Most interesting, it estimates the total number of cases per serving of that food eaten. THAT is the data I wanted.
>
> As we can see, unpasteurized milk is actually the fourth highest risk for listeria illness. . . . However, take a note that the *highest* risk is deli meats, which have ten *times* the rate of listeria illness per food serving. . . . To put that in perspective, for every serving of deli meat you eat, you have a *ten times greater risk* of getting sick from listeria than from drinking a glass of raw milk. However, one should note that raw fluid milk has a seven times greater illness per serving rate than pasteurized fluid milk does. So there is increased risk compared to pasteurized milk. But compared to deli meats—which are served without question millions of times a day in restaurants, grocery stores, and Yankee Stadium—raw milk is only 10% as dangerous on a per serving basis.
>
> In summary, according to that chart, cold hot dogs, deli meats, and pâté have a higher risk on a per serving basis for contracting listeria illness than drinking raw milk. Smoked seafood (like lox, from bagels and lox) and pre-cooked shrimp have about the same rate as raw fluid milk.
>
> So why is everyone up in arms about drinking raw milk? Especially when the rate of illness (at least for listeria) is TEN TIMES GREATER for deli meats!

You're putting your children at a TEN TIMES greater risk for contracting listeria by giving them a bologna sandwich for lunch than by giving them a glass of raw milk!!!

Greg also calculated, based on the same chart, that raw milk accounts for about 5 percent of all milk served, which would mean that around fifteen million Americans are raw milk drinkers. That seems pretty high, given estimates by Sally Fallon Morell of the Weston A. Price Foundation that there are somewhere between five hundred thousand and one million raw milk drinkers in the United States. With a population of about three hundred million, even one million raw milk drinkers would still only represent one-third of 1 percent of all Americans.

Actually, the real number is likely somewhere in between these two estimates. According to a 2002 survey of consumers in nine states (California, Georgia, Maryland, Minnesota, New York, Connecticut, Oregon, Tennessee, and Colorado) by a CDC-led consortium, the percentage of raw milk drinkers varies between 2.5 and 4. Extrapolating nationally, this translates into an impressive seven million to twelve million raw milk consumers. Interestingly, the percentage is about the same in California and Connecticut, where raw milk is sold in retail outlets, as it is in Maryland, where it is illegal (many raw milk drinkers travel to neighboring Pennsylvania for their milk). Even more interesting, consumption increases as incomes and education levels decrease, possibly reflecting the fact that farm workers tend to be heavy consumers of raw milk, and also produce soft raw milk cheeses. And consumption is highest among Asians, Hispanics, and "Other" racial groups—likely reflecting cultural traditions—versus whites.[21]

All this analysis left me convinced that, while raw milk can lead to foodborne illness, it is much less of a danger than the FDA and other public health agencies would have us believe. Yet I had trouble following along with the view among many committed raw milk drinkers that even the data showing modest danger from raw milk is way overstated. This view is personified by Sally Fallon Morell, president of the Weston A. Price Foundation, who feels that many reported illnesses linked via significant evidence by investigators to raw milk have been done so erroneously.

It's possible to get a flavor of how Fallon Morell and the foundation tend to view reported incidents of illness by reviewing one of the cases I mentioned at the outset of this book—the case of Dee Creek Farm in Washington State. At least eight members of a cow share run by Dee Creek were sickened, and the state's agriculture officials found evidence of pathogens in milk and manure samples from the farm that matched up with those found in ill consumers—evidence that is about as conclusive as it gets in the world of food-borne illness, akin to DNA evidence linking a suspect to a crime.

In a lengthy report about the Dee Creek case from the foundation, the section "Many Questions" discusses assorted alternative theories for how raw milk drinkers might have become ill. It points to another outbreak elsewhere in the state, noting that there had been additional outbreaks of illness from *E. coli* O157:H7 over the previous fifteen years, and that irrigation water sprayed on vegetables can contain *E. coli* O157: H7, among other possible explanations for the shareowners' illnesses. The foundation report says that state officials "ignored many facts that call their conclusions into question."[22]

The foundation's reluctance to admit to the likelihood that people can become ill from raw milk has led to a number of bitter debates among devoted raw milk drinkers. One such debate has revolved around the view held by some raw milk consumers, that the reason the rate of illnesses from drinking raw milk is so much lower than what's reported by public health authorities is that pathogens can't survive in raw milk that comes from pasture-fed cows.

This viewpoint was fueled by a 2002 study on raw milk that had been inoculated with pathogens; the scientific tests were conducted by a laboratory hired by Mark McAfee, the owner of Organic Pastures Dairy Co. Mark and others suggested that this report showed that most of the pathogens had died off in the raw milk. This study has since become part of the lore of the raw milk movement. But then someone on my blog posted a segment of the report saying that a significant number of pathogens had not only survived, but remained present in the milk for at least several days.

Do pathogens actually become overwhelmed by the "good" bacteria, the lactic acid, of grass-fed raw milk? This is a major bone of scientific contention that extends even beyond the raw milk community.

On one side, we have people like Pumendu Vasavada of the University of Wisconsin, who completely rejects that idea. In February 2009, at the International Association for Food Protection symposium on raw milk, he argued that raw milk is inherently dangerous because "it is a hospitable substrate" for pathogens. Vasavada also rejected the idea that "good bacteria" are beneficial. "Almost any bacterial species is capable of producing intestinal symptoms if swallowed in sufficient numbers," he stated.

At the other end of the spectrum, some raw milk advocates have argued that raw milk from cows raised on grass is a terrible medium for pathogens. Naturopath Ron Schmid stated in the first edition of *The Untold Story of Milk* that "the good bugs the cows naturally harbor are able to kill off potential pathogens such as salmonella and *E. coli* O157."

Mark McAfee seems to have backed off his claim posted on the Weston A. Price site, telling me, "With raw milk by itself, you don't see the explosion of bacteria. . . . Lactic acid producing bacteria is the safety mechanism that inhibits the growth of the bacteria." And a revised edition of *The Untold Story of Milk* eliminates most of the account of the study.

The results of the lab study that Organic Pastures commissioned really fall somewhere in between the original claims and what Professor Vasavada argues. BSK lab inoculated a huge number of cells into the OPDC milk, and then tested to see if the bacteria would grow, die, or stay the same over the shelf life at refrigeration temperatures. The data show that, overall, the number of bacteria stayed the same for these *E. coli* O157:H7 and *Listeria monocytogenes,* and declined sharply for salmonella.

A separate study I located from 1982 shows that campylobacter in both raw and sterile milk died off over the course of the refrigerated shelf life. Thus, neither raw nor highly pasteurized milk served as a favorable medium for this pathogen.

The bottom line appears to be that pathogens don't thrive in raw milk, but they don't all necessarily die off sufficiently to ensure certain consumers can't become ill.

As I editorialized on my blog:

> To me, the flareup of this debate is further evidence of the ideological nature of the struggle over raw milk. One side or the other uses partial data to press its case—raw milk is dangerous, or raw milk isn't dangerous. What this says to me is something I've said before, which is that it is possible to become ill from pathogens in raw milk, just as it's possible to become ill from pathogens in spinach and hamburgers. Raw milk isn't any more dangerous than many foods we consume that aren't subject to debate.
>
> It's time for us to move on to new avenues of exploration— maybe an updated and more complete version of the studies posted here. Or completely new studies. . . . Let's use ongoing illnesses to learn more about other possible determinants of food-borne

> illness—perhaps flavorings or colorings or sweeteners or whatever in seemingly ordinary foods; or genetic predisposition; or ongoing variations in individual immunity. Let's expand our thinking, instead of looking for ever more elusive "gotchas."[23]

Raw milk proponents have another answer to data and reports showing that people do become ill from raw milk. They argue that any dangers from infection by pathogens can be reduced significantly by regularly consuming raw milk, thereby building up immunity. They point to a 1987 study of thirty-one freshman fraternity pledges who, in the fall of 1982, went on a retreat to a large dairy farm owned by the parents of one member. Over the next ten days, nineteen of the thirty-one students developed gastrointestinal illness and were found to have campylobacter, a common source of food poisoning. Three others without symptoms were also found to be infected. Interestingly, ten individuals who consumed the tainted milk and showed no signs of illness or infection—a few students and some farmhands—were found to be regular consumers of raw milk.

The message? According to the study's authors: ". . . the attack rate (of campylobacter) was high among those exposed who had never previously consumed raw milk . . . this investigation confirms the presence of [*Campylobacter jejuni*] antibodies in persons chronically exposed to raw milk, and for the first time, to our knowledge, shows an association between high antibody levels and immunity to infection under field conditions."[24]

Mark McAfee of Organic Pastures cited this 1987 study on my blog following an outbreak of illnesses in Colorado from campylobacter in April 2009. He summed up its meaning this way: ". . . if you drink raw milk, with its biodoversity of good beneficial bacteria, your immune system will improve and you can feel much more confident that if a bad bug does come along . . . you will be much safer and probably immune to it because you have made a habit of eating its cousin in your cup of delicious raw milk. That is exactly what I tell people all day long. Raw milk consumption is a conscious deliberate effort to improve immunity and health."

He added, "Remember that the cleanliness of milking is a very small part of overall raw milk safety. The bigger and more important part is making sure that the environment of the cows is producing pathogen-free manure, etc. You want the right bugs in the corrals and pens and pastures. That's what is missing so often. Milking is not a sterile process . . . nor should it be."

In other words, regular consumption of raw milk reduces the chances you'll get sick, even if pathogens are present.[25]

The notion that Mark was denigrating the importance of sanitation prompted a regulator type who frequents my blog under the pseudonym Lykke to observe, "I'm all for grass-fed and pasture-based systems and preferentially buy animal products raised in non-confinement operations . . . however, it is not a replacement for cleanliness and sanitation when producing a raw food."[26]

Like so much in the world of raw milk, what you see isn't always what you get. While raw milk may at one time have been terribly dangerous, it isn't in this day and age, at least statistically speaking. That is because of the virtual elimination of brucellosis and bovine tuberculosis—the raw milk killers of the past—from the US cattle population. Modern raw milk dairies routinely test their cattle for these horrific diseases to ensure these bacteria are not shed in the milk.

Unlike today's four major food-borne illnesses (listeria, salmonella, *E. coli* O157:H7, and campylobacter) that most often get into the milk from sanitation problems, brucella and *Mycobacterium bovis* actually infect and create illness in the cows, and are shed in the cow's (or goat's) milk. Unfortunately, there aren't good treatments for either of these diseases once they hit humans. That rarely happens anymore, but because of the danger such diseases posed many years ago, the matter of raw milk's potential danger remains a highly emotional matter. And that emotional component is a major theme of the next chapter.

CHAPTER NINE

E. coli O157:H7 and the Education of Mary McGonigle-Martin

I've always found it intriguing that my introduction to the food-borne illness issue should have occurred in September 2006, when both bagged spinach and raw milk came under a cloud in California. Probably because I'm a reporter, I appreciate the detective work that must go into tracking down the pathogens that make people ill, whether from raw milk or some other food.

As it happened, two cases of illness growing out of the spinach and raw milk episodes capture key elements of the public health dilemma—unfortunately in a tragic way—when people become seriously ill from food, especially when they are children.

Before we look at these cases, though, we need some background information about food-borne illness. Most cases of food poisoning are discrete, anonymous affairs. People affected become moderately ill, then, when they are feeling better, they return to school or work. Few persons outside the victims' own communities of family, friends, and medical personnel are even aware that the illnesses have occurred.

So it is when seventy-six million Americans, or one out of every four people, contract food-borne illness each year, by the CDC's estimate. Nobody much cares when so many people are getting stomach upset here and there. It's a little like the common cold—we don't pay too much attention to it, because we know that we and our friends or neighbors will invariably get better in a few days.

But just as a few cases of the cold degenerate into bronchitis and pneumonia, so too do some cases of food-borne illness degenerate into something far more dangerous—conditions like hemolytic uremic syndrome (kidney failure) and Guillain-Barré syndrome (temporary paralysis), or worse.

Out of the 76 million estimated cases of food-borne illness each year, some

325,000 individuals are hospitalized, and 5,200 die. The majority of these deaths are from unknown causes or from noroviruses, which are passed around not only via food but also via person-to-person contact. The CDC figures that about fourteen million of the cases are attributable to "known pathogens" like campylobacter and salmonella, and these lead to sixty thousand hospitalizations and eighteen hundred deaths.[1]

What those data, with all the estimates and unknowns, say to me is that there is a lot we don't fully understand about food-borne illness—much more than I ever imagined. Before encountering the dubious cases of illness ascribed to raw milk that I described in chapter 2, I had imagined that public health authorities are able to quickly "connect the dots" and figure out what goes wrong.

In actuality, when victims suspect they have consumed bad food from the supermarket or restaurant, they may call their local public health department to request an investigation. In such cases, public health workers typically fill out a questionnaire that seeks to home in the actual symptoms, when the symptoms started, and what foods were consumed when. But unless a number of people from one area report similar symptoms, or several people become very ill, these reports typically remain buried in some files.[2]

Now, raw milk would not seem to be a big part of the apparent plague of food-borne illness we've heard so much about in recent years. As I pointed out in the previous chapter, data from both the CDC and the Center for Science in the Public Interest show anywhere from a few dozen to a few hundred illnesses attributed to raw milk consumption each year, with the average being under a hundred annually. Even allowing for the "multiplier effect" cited by public health experts, the numbers are still no more than the very low thousands.[3]

Okay, now it's time to return to the stories of the two children I mentioned at the start of this chapter. It seems that whenever there is a serious outbreak of food-borne illnesses, it results in one of two outcomes.

Sometimes, the authorities are able to make a connection between a sick individual and the actual cause of illness. So, as upsetting as the illness is, at least the individuals affected can gain some sense of relief and closure from learning about the source. Such was the situation in a case involving a young Ohio girl, who became seriously ill from contaminated spinach in September 2006.

But in other instances the authorities can't make a definitive connection between sick individuals and the ultimate cause. They may make an "epidemiological" connection—a circumstantial case based on a group of individuals who consumed the same food from the same source (say, everyone ate hamburgers from a single fast food outlet)—without being able to find any evidence of contamination at the producer's operation. The lack of a "smoking gun" can create all kinds of unresolved arguments and emotions about what happened and why. So it was with the second case of illness, in which a young California boy became just as seriously ill as the Ohio girl. In this case, though, the suspected culprit was raw milk. This case serves as a vivid reminder, not only of the difficulties of pinpointing cause, but also of how much more passion and emotion are stirred up when raw milk is suspected as the culprit.

The Case of Ashley Armstrong

The first case was that of Ashley Armstrong, the two-year-old daughter of Elizabeth and Michael Armstrong. The Ohio case was highlighted in a CNN broadcast as part of a "special investigation" by the network's chief medical reporter, Dr. Sanjay Gupta.

In late August 2006, after eating a dinner of lasagna and fresh spinach salad, Ashley and her older sister became ill. The sister had the symptoms of an upset stomach and recovered within a few days, but little Ashley just got sicker and sicker. After several days, she had blood in her stool, and shortly after arriving at a hospital's emergency room, her vomiting became progressively more serious. The culprit was identified as *E. coli* O157:H7, that especially dangerous aberrant of normally harmless *E. coli* bacteria.

Before long, the symptoms had become life threatening. According to Dr. Gupta, "Ashley's kidneys were failing and her brain swelling from a medical complication called hemolytic uremic syndrome or HUS." She was placed on kidney dialysis.

"HUS occurs in about 10 percent of small children with *E. coli* poisoning. It's most common in the young and the old," Gupta noted.

For several weeks, Ashley teetered between life and death. Although she finally turned a corner toward survival, it still wasn't until early December that she was well enough to return home from the hospital.

Even though she was home, she wasn't entirely healed. According to Gupta, "Life will never be the same. Ashley has to take a half dozen medications every day to treat her kidneys and related high blood pressure." A medical expert interviewed on the show predicted that her kidneys never would return to normal, and that she'd probably need a kidney transplant within three to ten years.

Ashley's father made the poignant observation that because Ashley would have to take powerful immunosuppressants to handle the kidney transplant, "It's quite unlikely she'll ever be able to have a kid of her own, to be pregnant."

Ashley's mother said she was so nervous that she avoided serving green vegetables to the family any longer. So most of what they ate were white foods.

The *E. coli* O157:H7 that made Ashley so ill also sickened about two hundred other people around the country. Three failed to recover, and died.

"It's amazing," said Michael Armstrong, "all this from a contaminated piece of spinach in a different state. It's kind of mind boggling."

The CNN program also described how California and federal authorities had launched a huge investigation to locate the source of the *E. coli* O157:H7 once it became clear in September 2006 that a national outbreak was in progress.

I was fortunate to learn about that investigation directly from one of the persons involved. I made a number of remarks on my blog from the fall of 2006 into early 2007, to the effect that the spinach and raw milk investigations were handled much differently, with the raw milk investigation being more intensive than the spinach investigation. Not so, argued Michele Jay-Russell, then a research scientist with the California Department of Health Services (now with the Western Institute for Food Safety), who sent me a publication on the outbreak.[4]

In an interview, she explained how a team of about a dozen investigators from the California Department of Health Services and the US Food and Drug Administration had gradually narrowed their search—based on tracking back several bags of Dole spinach recovered from sick consumers to various farms where the spinach was grown, in the lush and hilly San Benito and Monterey Counties in California's Central Coast region. The team lived for more than a month at a nearby hotel, spending their days collecting animal droppings, tracking pigs and cattle, and following runoff water in fields in the area.

By October, they had isolated four fields where the problem spinach might have been grown. Eventually, it all came down to one field, on leased land from Paicines Ranch in San Benito County. Ironically, the setting wasn't anything like what some raw milk advocates imagined. For example, a newly revised edition of *The Untold Story of Milk* by Ron Schmid reported on the spinach outbreak and its overlap with the raw milk illnesses, stating, "Several companies voluntarily recalled their spinach as the industry scrambled to find ways to prevent future outbreaks.... But the problem is complex. If, as most investigators suspect, runoff water from confinement farms is a source of the organism, it will be a continuing source of infection ..."[5]

Actually, the pathogen that caused the spinach outbreak was found in manure from grazing cattle a mile from the spinach field (cows that were being raised for grass-fed beef) that may have contaminated some river water, along with wild pigs, a regular nuisance, that had access to the spinach plantings, reported Jay-Russell. The details of the investigation are contained in a fifty-page report compiled by the California Department of Health Services and the FDA.[6]

A key finding from the report's executive summary states: "Potential environmental risk factors for *E. coli* O157:H7 contamination identified during the investigation included the presence of wild pigs in and around spinach fields and the proximity of irrigation wells used for ready-to-eat produce to surface waterways exposed to feces from cattle and wildlife."

The California spinach farm where investigators eventually tracked down the *E. coli* O157:H7 wasn't fined, and its main penalty appears to have been an interruption of production while the investigation proceeded from September to December 2006. However, the spinach industry as a whole suffered losses from the nationwide recall of all fresh spinach. While various legislators and others demanded improved sanitation practices at spinach production facilities, there were never any calls to restrict the sales of bagged spinach once the source of the contamination had been tracked down.[7]

The Case of Chris Martin

During September 2006, there were about two hundred cases of illness attributed to bagged spinach, and six attributed to raw milk. But even a handful of illnesses from raw milk seem to inflame the passions of public health and medical types, along with ordinary consumers, way out of proportion to the actual scope of the problem. Probably the most passionate situation I have been witness to involved Mary McGonigle-Martin, mother of Chris Martin, whose personal journal of her son's illness I quoted from extensively in chapter 2.

I had spoken to Mary a couple of times around the time I posted her hospital journal on my blog. She sounded like a very bright and cheerful woman. She was forty-eight when I first spoke with her in early 2007, and told me she was a high school guidance counselor in Southern California. Her husband, Tony, taught high school government and economics.

As I described in chapter 2, Chris Martin became sick in early September 2006 with bloody stools, seemingly endless diarrhea, and then failing kidneys from hemolytic uremic syndrome. He had to go on dialysis, and then hovered through seemingly interminable days and nights between life and death as his parents watched helplessly. He recovered well enough to return to his home in Marietta, California, in early November. Doctors, however, warned his parents that within ten years Chris could well experience serious kidney problems, leading to the necessity for a transplant.

While doctors suspected the culprit in Chris's illness to be *E. coli* O157:H7, they were never able to confirm the finding via stool samples. The best they could come up with was the diagnosis of HUS, a disease of the kidneys that often develops from shiga toxins, which are a potential complication from *E. coli* O157:H7 infection, when rapidly multiplying bacteria destroy red blood cells. The effects of HUS can be long-term and permanent.

In a note she wrote me, here is how Mary McGonigle-Martin recalls the doctors describing the potentially deadly effects of HUS:

All *E. coli* O157:H7/HUS cases, regardless of the source of contamination, look quite similar. The outcome is the same—permanent kidney damage is a given. The filters have been damaged. It's just a matter of time as to when kidney problems will appear. Each person is born with about one million of these filters. When a person reaches the 500,000 mark, the kidneys can't work properly. Our son, Chris, lost maybe 300,000 filters, so his kidneys are still working OK. But over time, the filters can't compensate. The kidneys weren't designed to work with less filters. They begin to operate like a water balloon. With use over the years, they will become larger and thinner and then they will begin to die. This is why kidney disease becomes inevitable. It will happen to Chris someday, we just can't predict the timeframe in which it will happen. Will he be 20, 30, or 40?

At the point the kidney loses enough of its filtering capacity, patients must go on dialysis, requiring that they have their blood mechanically filtered two or three times a week for six or eight hours at a time. It ties a person down, and is psychologically constraining—it's nearly impossible, for example, to take a long trip without arranging for dialysis along the way. Dialysis patients can sign up to receive a kidney from a cadaver, but that process can easily take two or three years. And the donated kidney usually doesn't last forever—perhaps 15 years, all the while requiring the patient to take various immune-suppressing drugs.

If the cases of Ashley Armstrong and Chris Martin sound similar in terms of illness symptoms and prognosis, it's because they are. HUS is a terrible disease, whether the E. *coli* O157:H7 that typically causes it comes from raw spinach or from raw milk.

But there was one big difference between the Ashley Armstrong and Chris Martin cases: The genetically matching E. *coli* O157:H7 that sickened Ashley had been tracked by investigators to specific spinach fields in California.

The story was much different, and more complicated, for Chris Martin. Of six children thought by California public health authorities to have become ill from raw dairy products—because they were all assumed to have consumed dairy products from Organic Pastures Dairy Co.—he was the only one who didn't have the E. *coli* O157:H7 in any stool samplings. But even allowing that he was sickened by the same genetically distinct E. *coli* O157:H7 that had triggered illness in the other five children, there were problems. While their E. *coli* O157:H7 was genetically the same, and also distinct from that found in spinach victims such as Ashley Armstrong, their E. *coli* strain couldn't be matched with any particular raw milk, or any producer of raw milk.

Investigators from the California Department of Health Services and the California Department of Food and Agriculture descended on Organic Pastures Dairy Co. in Fresno with as much intensity as those who scoured the spinach fields. They were saved much of the initial investigative work of the spinach team by virtue of the fact that only two dairies produce raw milk in California, and the milk the children had in common was from Organic Pastures.

While the raw milk report that the California Department of Health Services produced five months later is much slimmer than that completed in the spinach investigation—six pages total (four pages listing the officials who received copies and only two pages of text) versus fifty pages in the spinach investigation—it suggests a significant effort. It reports that on October 31, 2006, "fecal samples from 199 dairy cows were collected," and on November 6 another 163 fecal samples were taken from calves and non-milk-producing cows.

Perhaps the reason the raw milk report is so slim is that the investigators failed to find the matching *E. coli* O157:H7—the proverbial smoking gun. They did find *E. coli* O157:H7 in three cows, but they weren't matches for what was found in the children. And while the report isn't specific about the cows, Mark McAfee says the *E. coli* O157:H7 was found in nonmilking cows, and thus wouldn't have posed any danger to milk drinkers.

Even though investigators never tracked the pathogens that likely sickened Chris Martin and definitely sickened five other children to Organic Pastures Dairy Co., or anywhere else, the case became something of a political football. California's Department of Health Services concluded in its brief report, "Despite not finding the outbreak strain at this dairy, the source of infection for these children was likely raw milk products produced by the dairy." The conclusion was driven by what scientists refer to as "epidemiological evidence," or what most of us would refer to as circumstantial.[8]

Both raw milk advocates and critics used the results of this report to make their cases. As I described in chapter 3, John Sheehan, head of the FDA's Division of Plant and Dairy Food Safety, used the state's conclusion to bolster his argument that Maryland should maintain its ban on raw milk.

At the other end of the raw milk political spectrum, the Weston A. Price Foundation argued that nothing had been proven. Indeed, on its Web site, it tried in an October 2006 posting to connect the cases of the six ill children to the spinach outbreak.

> Organic Pastures Dairy Company (OPDC) raw milk products are back on the shelves following a recall in September. The recall occurred during the midst of the spinach contamination scare and seemed to be aimed at deflecting attention from the huge problems of *E. coli* O157:H7 contamination in produce. The state claimed that five raw milk-drinking children became ill, two of whom were hospitalized, given antibiotics and almost died. (The other three received no antibiotics and recovered quickly.) The mother of one child denied the illness had anything to do with raw milk and the other child had consumed spinach two days before the illness.[9]

That last sentence, in particular, deeply offended Mary McGonigle-Martin. She had told Mark McAfee, the owner of Organic Pastures, when he visited

Chris Martin in the hospital in September, that her son had consumed spinach, but that was before she knew all the facts in the case—specifically, that the spinach Chris consumed came from an open grocery bin, while the spinach contaminated with *E. coli* O157:H7 had been bagged before shipping to stores. She felt he took her early statement out of context, and that the Weston A. Price Foundation used his account of the conversation and followed suit.

The political and legal fault lines in this case had begun to be drawn. The failure of public health officials to make a direct connection between *E. coli* O157:H7 and raw milk created a level of uncertainty that made it impossible for Mary and her husband, Tony, to simply resume their previous lives. Some four months after Chris returned home from the hospital, they began to seek answers and express their opinions as to why their only child had nearly died—with much of their soul searching occurring on my blog.

Tony Martin joined a discussion on my blog in late March 2007 about whether children should consume raw milk:

> I have only one son. My wife and I gave him every advantage humanly possible from birth with regard to his diet—100% organic. At age seven, he was extremely outgoing, healthy, and happy. On Monday of Labor Day weekend (06) he is jumping into our pool with friends and having a blast. He drinks raw milk on Tuesday, and by Thursday is being admitted into the hospital with blood in his stool. Within one week, he is intubated, lifeless, in danger of heart failure as his tiny heart is beating 180 beats per minute, receiving kidney dialysis, and is only two weeks away from a brain seizure. Five children were sickened that weekend and the only common denominator among all five was raw milk, according to news accounts.
>
> So, if anyone out there would like to roll the dice and give their children raw milk, that is your right. I only hope you can live with yourself if you find yourself 24/7 at your child's bedside for 8 weeks praying he or she doesn't die.[10]

A couple of weeks later, Mary provided a highly personal account of what the experience of reliving Chris's experience via my blog had been like:

> I found The Complete Patient website when I was doing a search on raw milk. I was quite surprised to read a blog that was discussing

Lauren and Melissa Herzog and our children's e-coli story. This was on March 20, 2007.

It's been an emotional 19 days. Many nights I did not sleep well. Reliving our story has been challenging, but I believe it is a story that needs to be told. Tony and I suffered from post-traumatic stress as a result of our terrifying near-death experience with our son. Our favorite nephrologist was very concerned about our emotional health. He told us that what we experienced was horrific and the length of time we were in the hospital in a heightened state of anxiety would have an effect on us.

Mary went on in her commentary to recount how her belief in God had helped sustain her.[11]

The emotional accounts from Mary and Tony prompted the mother of Lauren Herzog, the second child who had become seriously ill, to join the discussion as well. Lauren was thought by her mother, Melissa, to have become ill after being served raw milk in a smoothie prepared by the girlfriend of her divorced husband while Lauren was spending a weekend with her dad. So there was a potentially explosive family situation compounding all the uncertainty about what actually made Lauren ill. For the purposes of this chapter, I have omitted most of the comments from Melissa Herzog, since her involvement was more emotional, and less focused, than Mary's. Melissa was certain the raw milk had made her daughter sick, that her ex-husband shouldn't have allowed Lauren to be served the milk, and that Mark McAfee was at serious fault—case open and shut.

The more searching and probing observations of Tony and Mary drew a range of responses from other readers of my blog. While most readers sympathized with these traumatized parents, a number with medical expertise tried to steer the conversation away from pure fear of pathogens and toward a more complete understanding of their role in our systems. Suzanne posted this explanation:

I have to add something to this discussion about raw milk "making" one sick because it gets to a point so incredibly fundamental to our health and understanding it.

As you know, bacteria and microbes are just opportunists. They will only make you sick when there is susceptibility or an underlying dysfunction to clean up. That is their role, and it is a profoundly important one from an evolutionary perspective. So getting sick is a crucial part of getting well in many cases, as getting sick, mounting a successful recovery, and then getting well again is the ultimate and original detox. It's how our bodies slough off imbalances and impurities.

And, yes, the antibiotics in this case absolutely inhibited this young boy's recovery. Getting the doctors to admit that is impossible, because allopathic medicine is based on the whole germ theory model, and antibiotics (and vaccines) are at the core of that paradigm, and thus constitute the third rail of western medicine as it exists today.

There are countless cases in the homeopathic literature about acute illness leading to profound and lasting improvements in the patient's load of chronic illness, in this case perhaps the ADD.

Looked at this way, as scary as it was, this illness may ultimately have benefited this child as a way for his body to retune its underlying imbalance.

I recognize this whole way of thinking is completely foreign in our culture, but it's a philosophy embraced by much of the rest of the world, and one I think we're slowly moving back to.[12]

Dave Milano, a frequent contributor to my blog, who works in the health care arena, had a bigger-picture view:

Raw-milk-related sicknesses are rare, generally minor, and self-limiting, and must be viewed in the context of other health factors, such as immune strength (which raw foods can improve) and, of course, collection techniques.

Perhaps today's typical American, indoctrinated by lawyers, government, vaccine manufacturers, doctors, and just about everybody else, into believing they can be protected from all hurtful things, cannot discuss these things sanely. Maybe that helps explain Mrs. Martin's awful sense of guilt ("I have to live with the fact that I gave my child raw milk that nearly killed him."). I do not mean to disparage Mrs. Martin in any way—can't say even that I wouldn't feel like her in similar circumstances. But I do believe that it is wrong to use her statements as a model. To do so would be to draw broad conclusions from narrow circumstances. That's bad science, and a bad way to run one's life. Mrs. Martin herself acknowledges that when she indicates that she would not prevent others from making their own minds up about raw milk.

The sane middle is where raw milk proponents will find success. It's where we all should want to be.[13]

The trauma Mary experienced, together with comments such as those I just quoted from Suzanne, and Dave Milano, drove Mary on an intensive search for the cause of her son's illness. The absence of a definitive explanation represented a huge puzzle she felt compelled to solve. She also had to face up to the reality that scientists don't fully understand the dynamics of food-based illness—the CDC's estimate of seventy-six million cases of foodborne illnesses each year is testament to that reality. So through the rest of 2007, Mary posted dozens of comments about how personally conflicted she was—as someone who was very careful about the food she and her family consumed, and concerned that no one else experience her family's pain. In late April, she stated:

> I quit eating red meat when I was 18 years old (thirty years ago). I read a few books about how cows are raised, fed, and killed. Add to that the amount of grain it takes to feed these animals, water to grow the grain (we could be feeding starving humans instead), and I decided it wasn't ethically responsible to eat meat from cows.
>
> Oh the irony that my child was almost killed from a bacteria created from these very cows. . . . My life philosophy is very aligned with yours. I do believe there is a larger picture at hand regarding our food supply in general; basically we're killing ourselves from the lack of nutrition, and that's not even touching upon the subject of pesticides, heavy metal, etc. . . . in our food supply.
>
> And yes, life is full of risks and you never know when something bad is going to happen. There are things you can control and there are things you can't. I believe you can and should control whether milking cows producing raw milk are contaminated with O157:H7. I think it would be as simple as checking the poop of each cow monthly/bi-monthly. Even if that raised the price of milk by a dollar a half-gallon, people would be willing to pay the price for safe milk.
>
> So what I'm proposing is testing the cow and the milk. Mark McAfee's slogan could be "The Poop Doesn't Lie!" He could post

the findings of his poop checks and advertise his milk as *E. coli* O157:H7 free.

I'm having a little fun here, but *E. coli* O157:H7 is quite serious and should be controlled as much as humanly possible . . .[14]

In response, several readers emphasized that the challenge was more complex than Mary had stated it, and that *E. coli* O157:H7 isn't passed on from a cow into the milk. Rather, it is contained in a cow's manure, and thus contaminates milk via manure getting into the milk, as Steve Bemis noted:

I'm troubled by what seems to be a missing link in the discussion. *E. coli* O157:H7 gets into milk by means of contaminated poop OUTSIDE THE ANIMAL. It doesn't somehow migrate into the milk by some internal metabolic, digestive or other process. Very simply, it's a hygiene issue where fecal contamination occurs after milking. Hence, it could even be a cross-contamination where fecal matter from one animal gets into the previously-clean milk taken from another. Or, contamination could occur from some other source entirely in the distribution chain through handling. Contamination of raw or pasteurized milk could occur in one's kitchen from contaminated spinach. I'm not pointing fingers here; just trying to clarify *how E. coli* gets into foods like milk. It's a physical process where the food comes into contact with the source of contamination. Some milk problems come with the milk, and come from the cow, like bovine Johnes which is much more likely in the real world, which can in turn cause Crohn's [disease] in humans, and which by the way, is not destroyed by pasteurization.[15]

Mary would not be so easily assuaged, responding to Steve:

I get that Steve. My point is that *E. coli* O157:H7 can't get on the outside (by pooping) and then into the milk if it's not on the inside of the cow first.

After all the testing last October at Organic Pastures farm, one milking cow out of around 300 had *E. coli* O157:H7. [*Author's note:* Although it was not clear from the state report that a milking cow had *E. coli* O157:H7.] It's almost a perfect herd, but not perfect enough. One cow with e-coli can do damage.

Since *E. coli* O157:H7 was not originally found in nature (it is something that developed/mutated because of all the modern farming practices), I don't think it should be allowed to exist in a milking cow's colon, if this cow is producing raw milk. I personally think the risk is too high. It's a disaster waiting to happen and I'm not sure every dairy can be clean enough all the time to prevent its possible contamination.

If all cows are clean on the inside, there can't be e-coli contamination.[16]

Miguel, a dairy farmer and cheesemaker, added to Steve Bemis's point by offering a natural preventive approach to becoming sick from *E. coli* O157:H7:

E. coli O157:H7 have absolutely no way to tell if they are inside of a cow or a human. If they can mutate from common e-coli inside a cow, they can surely do so inside a human. The key to protecting yourself against this bacteria, whether it enters your system on some food or occurs spontaneously as a result of common e-coli mutating, is to maintain an internal environment that is hostile to *E. coli* O157:H7. This bacteria proliferates in an acid environment (grain-fed cattle or for that matter grain-fed children), an environment where other friendly bacteria have been suppressed by antibiotics or food preservatives (which are antibiotics—that's why they preserve food).[17]

In a later comment, Miguel offered Mary a further assessment as to why food-borne illness is a bigger problem today than it was fifty or seventy-five years ago:

Think for a moment about how food has changed since our grandparents were young.

Back then producing and preserving food was a big part of the local economy. Much of the food they consumed only traveled a few miles to get to their plate. Much of it came directly from farms to households. Still, it needed to be preserved for the winter. They preserved the food by fermenting it. Fermentation is a biological process. Bacteria was the essential ingredient in this food. People ate fermented food every day. Sauerkraut, cultured butter, pickled beets, even ham and sausage were products of fermentation. . . . Spices, salt and smoking were used to ensure that the beneficial bacteria predominated. These foods are all examples of probiotics that people consumed daily.

Why can't we get our probiotics from those same foods today?

Today we live in a global economy. To be profitable food has to have a long shelf life. It has to travel hundreds or thousands of miles to get to your plate. To ensure the long shelf life, the bacteria have to go. All of the foods our grandparents ate as fermented foods are now pasteurized (canning is pasteurization) or irradiated. Pickles are made by adding vinegar rather than the old-fashion method of fermentation.

If the food production industry tried to sell us on pasteurization as a way to enable the industry to consolidate and operate on a global scale, would you buy that?

That is why they explain it as a way to make the food safe. And that is why they teach people to fear bacteria. Fear is a great motivator.[18]

Gradually, Mary's comments turned more pointed as she revealed examples of "evidence" she had obtained to help put the puzzle together.

During late April 2007, she reported that she had uncovered important information at California's Department of Health Services:

I talked to the person at the state department in charge of the investigation of possible e-coli contamination from Mark's farm. He told me they found *E. coli* O157:H7 in three cows. One was a milking cow and two were dry herd cows, but they were not the same blueprint as the e-coli found in the kids. And this answers my question as to why they were testing the cows . . . duh!!! They were trying to find the matching blueprint.

I also talked to Mark (before I talked to the person at the state) and he told me they found e-coli in 3 of his cows (he was shocked), but said they were all dry herd cows. So there is a conflict of information. I tend to believe the guy from the state department.[19]

During the summer of 2007, the debate intensified as Mark and Mary began to trade direct charges and countercharges on my blog.

In August, I sought to put the whole thing into perspective when Mark agreed to discuss the case and his frustration in trying to answer charges against him. I wrote:

> I've long been of two minds on the illnesses involving the Martin and Herzog children, which their parents attribute to raw milk. On the one hand, I appreciate the suffering they and their families went through—I think anyone who has children can appreciate how terrible it must have been. I can also understand the desire by Mary McGonigle-Martin and Melissa Herzog to get hard answers—make that final answers—as to what caused the illnesses, and also their frustration about slight changes in the explanations offered by Mark McAfee of Organic Pastures Dairy Co. as to what might have happened.
>
> On the other hand, I sometimes feel as if the whole search for "truth" in these two cases puts raw milk under a scrutiny that is way out of proportion to its role in food-borne illness in this country (where raw milk is merely a blip on the radar screen) . . . and that this blog contributes to that problem. The media don't do this kind of dissection when listeria in deli meats sickens people, but they do all kinds of headstands when ag officials say listeria was found in some farmer's raw milk, even when no one got sick.
>
> As I said, I can appreciate the frustration Mary McGonigle-Martin feels over what she sees as variations in Mark McAfee's explanation of what went on. So I called Mark and raised the issue with him.
>
> Basically, he didn't deny that his story may have changed a bit in the many re-tellings, but he seemed to say in response that how he explains what happened is irrelevant, since Organic Pastures has never been implicated in the problem.
>
> "After everything is said and done, California accused me, the parents accused me, and nothing was found. Did [Mary's] child have *E. coli* O157:H7? No. So what's the point? That's my point. And if you're going to say I made four kids sick, show me the bacteria" [that connects to Organic Pastures].
>
> He added, "My heart goes out to her [Mary]. She has the best of intentions. But the investigators did not find a connection. . . . She is passionately filled with wishful thinking. What can I say?"

To Mark, the entire experience . . . is indicative of a larger cultural problem in the US—our desire to find a culprit for whatever calamity we may be experiencing. "We are one of those countries that must have a diagnosis and figure out who's responsible for a problem and hang them. . . . Instead of looking at ourselves to build up our immune systems and exercise, instead we try to find 'them' and shoot 'them.'"

He added, "It's all about getting someone else to pay for your problem. It's always someone else's fault."

He also sees our culture excusing side effects and deaths from drugs, and not being nearly so forgiving for food. The growing problem of illness from disease-resistant bacteria in hospitals "is all excused because drugs cure and foods don't. It's the great distraction."

Is Mary being unreasonable in continually questioning a suspect who's essentially been cleared by the most intensive investigation the authorities can undertake—authorities, mind you, who came into the investigation wanting more than anything to hang the suspect? Is Mark being unreasonable in not wanting to be held accountable for his answers to accusations of something he's been cleared of, and instead wanting to talk about the bigger issues?[20]

Mary was quick to respond to my interview of Mark, posting three different comments on this one piece alone. In one, she bemoaned what she saw as Mark's lack of "respect":

I've been self-analyzing why I'm so bothered by Mark McAfee's statements. His dairy was cleared—no *E. coli* O157:H7 was found in any milk on the shelves, at his farm, or in his cows (with the same blueprint). So why does he have to exaggerate the story with false information? Why does he have to play the "victim" role?

He was not victimized. He benefited from all the media exposure. He is a shrewd businessman. His profits are up and he has more people drinking his milk than before the children became ill. In a recent article I read, it stated that Mark has a new distributor and he is making a jump from selling his milk in 300 stores to 500 stores. His business is booming, and I'm very happy for all the people who now have access to raw milk.

If he is 100% sure that his milk is not responsible for the children becoming ill then I believe he should show a little more respect to the suffering that these kids and families endured. He can show this respect by being honest about all the facts (what our kids ate) and details involved in the investigation of his farm (they didn't test all of his cows and they did find *E. coli* O157:H7 in one milking cow and two dry herd cows). He should not have a defensive response because I would want to know factual information about the blueprint pattern number of the sick children. This defensive response makes me think he knows this information to be true (his attorneys were able to obtain it).

It's disrespectful to our families to make statements that "it's wishful thinking" on my part because I'm trying to validate information. He's making these insensitive remarks because he thinks I'm going to use this information against him. He's behaving like a guilty person. Actions always speak louder than words.

When Mark came to Loma Linda Children's Hospital, he presented himself as a caring man who was trying to inform us of the true facts about all four of the sick children. He said the media was reporting false information. This is like calling the kettle black. He's now doing the same thing to benefit himself. Mark McAfee runs an amazing dairy but he seems to lack good character.

Then she became philosophical, exonerating Mark and instead blaming our society's tampering with nature for her experience:

Drinking raw milk from healthy cows is not inherently dangerous. There is an extremely small risk of drinking a batch that could be contaminated, and, in my opinion, far less a risk than eating a hamburger. . . . What caused Chris to become ill was *E. coli* O157:H7, not raw milk. I don't blame Mark McAfee. If his milk was somehow contaminated, it was not because of some negligence on his part. The bottom line is . . . life is not fair and sometimes bad things happen. Accidents happen. If he was a completely irresponsible dairy farmer, I'd have a different opinion. Raw milk dairy farmers are burdened with a huge responsibility, and Mark's perfect record proves that he takes numerous precautions in preventing pathogens from entering the raw milk he produces.

I believe OP raw milk is safe to drink. However, if some small batch of milk somehow became contaminated last year, I hope Mark brainstormed all the possibilities (how could this happen on a farm so scrutinized for pathogens) so it doesn't happen again. Mark's arrogant attitude toward government officials makes it hard to discern if he really believes his cows could "never" produce milk with pathogens. . . . To quote Ron Schmid (author of *The Untold Story of Raw Milk*), "But to expect or demand perfection from any dairy would be ludicrous, and any raw food may on occasion carry pathogenic organisms that may precipitate illness in susceptible individuals." . . .

My son became ill from some sort of "freak" bacteria that is a direct result from our sick farming methods. In order to quickly fatten up cows, they are fed a high-grain diet, which is not natural to their digestive system. They also live in inhumane conditions that put stress on their bodies. In order to prevent them from becoming ill, they're loaded up with antibiotics. This somehow created a perfect environment for bacteria to trade genetic material. We now have to live in world with shiga-producing e-coli. Thirty years ago this reality did not exist.

E. coli O157:H7 is symbolic of what we are doing to our world. We have tampered with nature and there is a price to be paid.[21]

As summer faded and the one-year anniversary of Chris's illness and hospitalization approached, a strange and ironic regulatory blip occurred. Inspectors with the CDFA said they had discovered *Listeria monocytogenes* in raw cream from Organic Pastures. This prompted Mary to recall the emotions surrounding the anniversary:

It was an eerie Labor Day weekend here in California. It was blazing hot just like last year. I couldn't help but think about all the people drinking raw milk produced in this heat. Are they vulnerable because it is so hot? Bacteria explode in the heat. I kept wondering, "Is there going to be another outbreak?" I'm glad to hear that so far no one has become ill and I do hope it is a "testing" flaw and not a real contamination problem.

This time last year we had been in the hospital for four days. Chris had non-stop painful diarrhea and vomiting. Today was the

day Chris started having pre-HUS symptoms—possible appendicitis or ulcerative colitis. This is when doctors became extremely
concerned. This is the day before our lives changed forever. Chris
was diagnosed with HUS on day five.

Tomorrow it will be a year since we were told that Chris had a
chance of dying simply because of ingesting a foodborne pathogen.[22]

And on it went. Each time the matter of children's illnesses came up, it
seemed the entire debate and counterdebate opened up between Mary and
those who thought she was raising the hysteria level for raw milk. During
this iteration of the debate, though, something unusual happened: Mark
McAfee interjected himself into the discussion.

In my experience as a business journalist, this was highly unusual, possibly
unprecedented. No business owner being accused of selling a tainted product
would ever discuss the details of the case with the affected consumer. Even
if he or she wanted to, no lawyer worth his salt would allow it to happen. Yet
Mark posted several lengthy comments reiterating many of the arguments
described previously in this chapter and other chapters, and Mary answered
each one with her version of events.

Finally, I decided the whole thing had become too personal and petty. I
suggested that Mary continue her research and investigation of what really
happened, and feel free to share it on my blog. If she still felt that some
other organization—Organic Pastures, a hospital, a doctor, the Weston A.
Price Foundation—was at fault, she should take advantage of our country's vast legal system staffed by more lawyers per capita than any country
in the world for pursuing cases of negligence, libel, medical malpractice,
and so forth. In other words, move on from the seemingly endless personal
accusations.

In early 2008, Mary and her husband filed suit against Mark and OPDC
in California state court, alleging that OPDC's milk had sickened Chris
Martin. (Melissa Herzog filed a nearly identical suit on behalf of her daughter Lauren.) When the suit was filed, Mary's lawyer advised her against
commenting on my blog, so her public comments ceased. He also advised
her against doing an interview with me in connection with this book, which
is why I have relied on her comments on my blog made before the suit.

Mary's suit against Mark McAfee included the report from the California
Department of Health Services on the state's investigation of the September
2006 outbreak of *E. coli* O157:H7 that assessed the circumstances of the

illness.[23] This was the first I had seen of the report, and I thought it was confusing in important respects, especially in light of the varying information Mary and others had posted on my blog about the circumstances surrounding the children's illnesses. Here is what I wrote on my blog about the report:

> The memo itself never identifies Organic Pastures by name, referring only to "Brand A dairy." ... [and concludes] that "the source of infection for these children was likely raw milk products produced by the dairy." ...
>
> There are a few other curiosities, one being the Health Services' depiction of the six children's illnesses: "Four patients drank raw milk regularly. One patient drank raw milk only once; he was served raw chocolate colostrum as a snack when visiting a friend. One patient denied drinking Brand A raw milk but his family routinely consumed Brand A raw milk."
>
> So, if I've got this right, five of the six ill children were confirmed drinkers of raw milk during the suspected danger period. And one of those five—Chris Martin—was never diagnosed with *E. coli* O157:H7. So really, we have four confirmed raw milk drinkers who had *E. coli* O157:H7—one-third of the children are already in doubt about what they consumed or what illness they had. Plus, the report suggests that a boy was the only one who drank raw milk only once, yet many times on this blog, Melissa Herzog said Lauren was served raw milk once while visiting her father (they were separated), and that otherwise she didn't drink raw milk. So now we have questions about a third illness, or half the children.
>
> If this thing isn't settled in advance of going to trial, I can see where the lawyers are going to have a field day trying to figure out who did what to whom, and when. And remember, the *E. coli* O157:H7 found in the five children was never picked up in all the many tests of animals and milk at Organic Pastures.
>
> I think the thing that has bothered me most about this whole matter, aside from the contradictory evidence and the lack of a "smoking gun," has been the fact that it feeds the long-time perception of raw milk as more dangerous than other foods, which we know from US Centers for Disease Control data to be untrue. Toward what end?[24]

The entire case became more complex as time went on. By April 2008, there was even a conspiracy theory of sorts being tossed about. Amanda Rose, an ardent California raw milk consumer, claimed in a lengthy analysis on her blog that she had figured out why California investigators were unable to find the offending pathogen during their investigation of Organic Pastures in September and October 2006.

She pointed to a statement the dairy's owner, Mark McAfee, made on his Web site, to the effect that raw colostrum sold by his dairy in September 2006 had been outsourced. (Colostrum is the nutrient-rich first milk produced by a mother for her calves in the days immediately after birth.) Technically, colostrum isn't even a dairy product, but rather under FDA rules is considered a nutritional supplement, and often sold in pill form.

Organic Pastures, however, sells raw colostrum as one of its products, and one of the six children whose illness from *E. coli* O157:H7 was blamed on raw milk had consumed colostrum, according to the state report. Because Mark McAfee admitted to obtaining his colostrum from an outside dairy— one that she said had questionable sanitation—Amanda Rose speculated that this may have been the source of the problematic *E. coli* O157:H7.

"From the consumer point of view, this particular nutritional supplement is produced in the mammary gland of a cow, gets dumped into the same sort of bottle with the same equipment, and it could well have carried the deadly pathogen strain in the 2006 recall," Amanda stated.[25]

In a comment on Amanda's blog, Mark McAfee said that "our deal was to purchase colostrum from first calf heifers that were pasture-grazed and organically certified. That is exactly what we did at that time. This is no secret. We have been open about this at all times." He said Organic Pastures discontinued such purchases when the outside dairy lost its organic certification.

This was certainly an interesting theory, but, unfortunately, we'll likely never know for sure whether the colostrum was contaminated and, if it was, whether it might have somehow infected milk produced at Organic Pastures. The CDFA conducted thorough tests of all Organic Pastures' equipment and came up with nothing.[26]

A blogger on my site, Kathryn, expressed a different kind of concern about the families' court suit: its effect on the children:

> I have seen, since the beginning of this *E. coli* breakout, a real fearful[ness] exhibited by Mary in general. It is hard to have a tragic occurrence, and not let it take over your life. But to have a healthy

emotional life, it is necessary to overcome those fears and reflect on a wholistic healing. I am sad for Lauren and Chris that they will be embroiled as victims for some time to come. Victimhood can create serious emotional disabilities in maturing youngsters, and it is a great burden to bear for a long time.[27]

Because Mary from the beginning struck me as an extremely decent and sensitive person, I worried about her pursuing a potentially bruising court case. She was so racked with guilt ("I'll always have to live with the fact that I almost killed my son," she stated at various times) and conflict (loyalty to both foodies and germophobes) and anger (at Mark McAfee of Organic Pastures and Sally Fallon Morell of the Weston A. Price Foundation) and fear (whether Chris will eventually need a kidney transplant), it was hard to imagine her dealing with a highly public case. Above all, I wondered if she'd ever be able to "let go."

The case pressed ahead, with theatrics impressive even by California standards, and Mary seemed not put off in the least—in fact, she seemed to thrive. In August 2008, Mary posted on YouTube a videotape of her son, Chris, on life support during September 2006. It shows him at various stages of his treatment, mostly breathing laboriously with tubes and needles connected to his arms and chest, and, at one point, with an oxygen mask over his nose and mouth.

What was interesting to me was that Mary had sent a copy of the same video to me about nine months earlier, with the understanding that I would keep it private. She wanted me to understand as fully as I could how traumatic her son's illness had been. It was difficult to watch the tape and not agree.

What had prompted Mary to post the video when she did was that California was in the midst of a legislative struggle over restricting certain raw milk standards, and Mary wanted to influence the debate so as to tighten standards. (I discuss the entire debate in detail in chapter 11.) But apparently, because her court suit had been filed months earlier, Mary some days later took down the YouTube video.

Through the winter of 2008–2009, testimony, known as depositions, was taken in the court suits filed by the Martin and Herzog families. Such testimony isn't open to the public, but the lawyer for the two families, Bill Marler of Seattle's MarlerClark, posted background about the cases from time to time. In mid-March, he posted lengthy background descriptions of the experiences of Chris Martin and Lauren Herzog.[28]

As I noted earlier in this chapter, the biggest hole in the case, from the initial reporting of illnesses in September 2006 when investigators turned Organic Pastures upside down looking for pathogens, was the absence of a direct link between the *E. coli* O157:H7 found in children who became ill and the dairy itself—a so-called smoking gun. In March 2009, Marler posted a document that he said plugged that hole of "identifying the causal connection" between Organic Pastures milk and the sick kids.[29]

The emotions that always seem to surround raw milk came out when I asked Bill Marler what the document's purpose was. He addressed my previously expressed skepticism about the linkage in his blog posting, answering "one of my fans" (me) by saying the document "was prepared by me and given to counsel for Organic Pastures and the grocery stores so they would better understand our position in the litigation. We have nothing to hide. I also told him [me] with respect to his version of the facts—'Obama could be a Muslim and the earth could be 5,000 years old. All possible, but very, very unlikely.'"[30]

So what was Marler's serious answer to my "version of the facts"? He offered the opinions of six "of the most respected leaders in the field of epidemiology."[31] The first one quoted, Dr. William Keene, an epidemiologist with the Oregon Public Health Division, went through a mathematical assessment of the probability of so many of the children who became ill being linked to Organic Pastures, and stated: "To put it in plain English, it is implausible that this association would occur by chance alone."

But Keene betrayed his prejudice against raw milk when he explained the supposed contamination of Organic Pastures' raw milk: "It's pretty much the same story over and over, there is no mystery in this process. Raw milk is virtually *always* contaminated with bovine feces, and the evidence indicates that Organic Pastures milk was no exception." This, of course, is a falsehood, based on evidence that unpasteurized *conventional* milk is often laced with pathogen-containing feces—he said as much when he noted that "there are traces of cow manure in pooled milk after collection . . ."

Given his apples-and-oranges comparison of Organic Pastures raw milk with conventional unpasteurized milk, it was difficult to accept Keene's nearly condescending explanation of why the pathogens in the sick children were never found at the Organic Pastures dairy. He told us that "O157 shedding by bovines can be very intermittent, such that positive samples on one day can be followed by negative samples for days or weeks thereafter. In summary, the lack of matching O157 culture results at the dairy is not at all inconsistent with the conclusion that Organic Pastures was the source. . . . Public health agencies do not have the resources to collect and test potential thousands of samples over a period of months to fully document the obvious." Well, at least it was obvious to Keene.[32]

Another expert, Michael Osterholm, a professor at the University of Minnesota's School of Public Health, explained:

> the lack of isolation of the outbreak strain of *E. coli* O157:H7 from the cattle on the farm is not unexpected. I know from previous outbreaks that a specific strain of *E. coli* O157:H7 may be transient in a bovine population. Unless investigators were sampling at the farm on the day or days of production associated with the outbreak case consumption it is possible to not detect that strain in the raw milk. In addition, it's possible the outbreak strain was in the milk on the day that investigators did sample but the presence of the organism was not uniform throughout the bulk tank or it was in levels not detectable by our current laboratory techniques due to the competition of other bacterial contamination (i.e., such as other fecal coliforms). The human gut is the ultimate bioassay and will tragically "detect even one or two *E. coli* bacterium" that then leads to infection.[33]

Osterholm's argument seemed both a candid admission about the limits of existing tracking techniques, and a questionable case for relying on circumstantial evidence. In other words, the fact that we lack the capabilities to find the culprit pathogens shouldn't stand in the way of placing blame.

Mark McAfee was understandably upset by the ongoing postings by the MarlerClark firm. Yet Mark and the Weston A. Price Foundation weren't totally innocent, either.

In a January 2008 press release, the Weston A. Price Foundation stated that "thorough investigation of the milk, the cows and even the manure at Organic Pastures Dairy failed to find virulent *E. coli* or any other pathogen" during the September 2006 investigation.[34] Yet the February 2007 report by the Department of Health Services said three cows were found to harbor the pathogen. It was a different strain than what sickened five of the six children, but it was, undeniably, a form of *E. coli* O157:H7.

Clearly, only a judge and jury, or perhaps a mediated settlement, could bring closure to this case.

CHAPTER TEN

When It Comes to Food, How Much Freedom Should We Have to Take Risks?

Just as 2006 was drawing to a close, with most people on break between Christmas and New Year's, an Ohio judge came down with a decision in the case I referred to in chapter 4 about Carol Schmitmeyer (see pages 60–63). Not only did he rule in her favor, but he castigated the Ohio Department of Agriculture over its handling of herd-share agreements.

Yet as winter turned into spring 2007, there remained considerable uncertainty about the highest-profile of the government's raw milk cases: that involving Richard Hebron in Michigan.

I felt privately as if the case against Hebron, the target of the sting operation the previous October (described in chapter 1), was going to turn out badly. Victor Fitz, the Cass County prosecutor, had been telling me in my periodic check-in phone calls that a big reason he was taking so long in deciding whether to prosecute was that he was tracking down leads in Pennsylvania, Indiana, and Missouri—from providers of products like beef and cheese and honey to the Ann Arbor cooperative Richard Hebron served. In my estimation, Fitz had spent too much time chasing down too many leads to simply drop the case.

However, in mid-March I had a discussion that, in retrospect, should have tipped me off to the direction the case was heading. I realized I didn't know much about Fitz, aside from the fact he was the prosecutor in this case, so during this March conversation I inquired into his professional background. He told me he was forty-nine years old and had spent much of his career as an assistant prosecutor, "where you do everything" in terms of cases.

Drug cases and homicides constituted the bulk of his experience, as both an assistant prosecutor and as chief prosecutor, he told me. Cases against producers of raw dairy products? "This is not routine," he said. "And I hope I don't have too many more of these going forward."

I didn't fully appreciate it at the time, but Fitz was telling me, in effect, that he wanted to be rid of this case. He didn't want the spectacle of a trial in which he was trying to convict a subsistence farmer of a felony, based on whether he should be distributing unpasteurized milk to mature adults who were seeking it of their own free will.

Had I grasped what Fitz was really saying, the news at the end of April would not have been as big a surprise as it was for me. Here is how I described it in a blog entry dated April 24, 2007:

> Six months after launching an elaborate sting operation against Michigan farmer Richard Hebron while he delivered raw milk to cow-share owners in Ann Arbor, and a follow-on investigation that spanned at least three other states from Pennsylvania to Missouri, Michigan walked away from the entire mess by giving the farmer little more than a slap on the wrist.
>
> You could almost hear authorities from Michigan's Department of Agriculture (MDA) and county prosecutor offices in Cass and Washtenaw counties breathe a sigh of relief this morning as they wrapped up the embarrassing case by agreeing to a settlement with Hebron whereby he can continue distributing raw milk to members of the Family Farms Cooperative and approving in principle the validity of cow-share agreements. In exchange, all Hebron needs to do is refrain from distributing raw milk through any retail establishment (which he hasn't been doing since the sting operation), "come into compliance" on a number of food preparation and processing matters on foods apart from raw milk, and pay a $1,000 "administrative fine," according to [Katherine] Fedder, head of the MDA's Food and Dairy Division.
>
> The MDA's soft and reasoned approach demonstrated today is a far cry from previous talk of a trial of Hebron on felony charges for supposedly violating state rules against sale of raw milk . . .
>
> Hebron, for his part, isn't overly ecstatic about the settlement. He not only lost about $7,000 of confiscated produce, but many thousands of additional dollars in revenues from people scared off by the government action. He says co-op sales have just in the last few weeks rebounded to pre-sting levels—driven in part by the media

attention to his case, as well as by a realization by some that "they haven't been eating as well, and are starting to see health issues return." But he worries about "six or eight regulations and codes they now want followed. . . . They want to get me under their thumb with all these regulations."[1]

Privately, I wondered if this case represented a turning point in the government's raw milk offensive, coming as it did just a few months after Ohio's new Democratic governor had ordered the state to refrain from appealing the Carol Schmitmeyer court victory in late 2006.

What had essentially happened within the space of five months was that two states in which the sale of raw milk was expressly forbidden had been turned around. Consumers could now legally obtain raw milk in Michigan and Ohio via so-called cow-share or herd-share agreements—legal agreements whereby consumers buy ownership shares in the cows for anywhere from $50 to a few hundred dollars. Then the consumers pay ongoing "boarding fees" to share in the cost of feeding and housing the animals, and in exchange receive some set amount of milk, typically a gallon or two each week. Individual farms might have one hundred or two hundred shareholders each. For individuals committed to consuming raw dairy products, herd shares were a great means of obtaining a regular supply of raw milk.[2]

Might the avalanche of publicity and testimonials that had apparently persuaded Michigan authorities to back off now persuade authorities in places such as New York, Pennsylvania, and California to do the same? Might the overseer of the war on raw milk producers, the FDA, perhaps be persuaded as well? I wanted to think so.

In retrospect, I didn't fully appreciate just how much resolve the regulators had. Because by early summer one of the most curious, and serious, cases in the entire raw milk struggle had just begun to unfold in upstate New York, on a ramshackle dairy farm run by a sincere and kindly couple, Barb and Steve Smith.

Like many of today's sustainable farmers, Barb and Steve Smith had left professional careers in the mid-1990s, while in their forties, to fulfill a personal vision of starting anew tending dairy cows on their own land. But like many newbie farmers, they found the road harder and harsher than they expected. They milked thirty cows and sold the milk the traditional way, through a processor that two or three times a week sent a tanker truck through their area to pick up milk from local farmers.

It's the way most dairy farmers sell their milk. The tanker truck shows up, empties the dairy's bulk tank storing milk from the previous day or two, and drives off. Some time later, after the processor tests the milk for bacteria counts and butterfat content, the farmers receive a report as to how much milk was taken, and the price that will be paid. If the total bacteria count is below a certain threshold, say two hundred thousand per milliliter, the farmer might receive a bonus over the regular rate. For organic milk as well, the price is usually higher than normal.

What made the life so difficult was the fact that the Smiths, like other dairy farmers, had to pay for feed and other expenses to maintain the cows in advance of being paid by the dairy processor. This was an especially difficult burden in winter, when the cows couldn't graze on pasture. "We had thirty cows, and we had to have $100,000 tied up," recalls Barb. "We used to borrow money to pay for the winter feed."

Compounding the stress was that the Smiths didn't have any control over the prices they received. The processor set those based on market prices for milk. If the Smiths didn't think the price was high enough, there wasn't another processor to go to, since everyone essentially paid the same. During the late 1990s, the Smiths might receive $15 per hundredweight of milk (each hundredweight is equal to a little over eleven gallons). For organic milk, the price could be $18 per hundredweight. This was on the order of $1.35 to $1.65 a gallon. By the time of the food commodity boom of the mid-2000s, farmers were doing much better, receiving $20 and more per hundredweight, or nearly $2 a gallon.

The problem facing the Smiths was the same problem facing owners of small dairies everywhere: The prices they received yielded little, if any, profit. In 1998, they did a calculation, and according to Steve, "We figured that with milk we were earning something like $1 an hour." Their little calculation helps explain why major dairy-producing states like Wisconsin, Kentucky, and Vermont have lost thousands of dairy farms in the years since World War II. The US Department of Agriculture reports that the number of farms with dairy cows fell by an astounding 88 percent between 1970 and 2006. And more than half of milk production now comes from dairies with more than five hundred cows, according to the USDA.[3]

There was one sliver of hope in the Smiths' situation. Beginning in 1995, they took advantage of a New York law that allowed the sale of unpasteurized milk directly from the farm, figuring that such sales might help supplement their income. At first, there was nothing to speak of, as they had only one regular customer taking advantage of the offer.

Gradually, though, the situation began to change as raw milk increased in popularity. The Smiths' farm was about an hour northwest of Ithaca, the home of Cornell University, and its community of more than twenty thousand students, faculty, and support staff. This community of educated professionals and students was becoming ever more interested in locally produced and nutrient-dense food, and raw milk filled the bill. By early 2007, the Smiths had between twenty and thirty customers traveling to their farm each week, generating about $1,500 a month in welcome additional income.

This growing trickle of customers always had two main complaints. First, they wanted a way to access the Smiths' milk more conveniently, without having to get into their cars and drive nearly two hours round trip. Second, they wanted additional raw milk products, like butter, cream, yogurt, and kefir. The raw milk permit granted to the Smiths, and a handful of other dairies around the state, not only required consumers to make their purchases at the farm but also limited the farmers to selling only raw milk, prohibiting the other raw dairy products consumers wanted.

The Smiths might have continued along this middle road that combined additional income with the state's limitations had it not been for one additional frustration that was thrown into the mix during 2006, just around the time the national campaign against raw milk producers was gearing up. That year, the New York Department of Agriculture and Markets implemented a more automated system of dairy inspections.

Dairy inspectors are like the police of the dairy farmers. They inspect dairies for cleanliness and adherence to certain regulations. The inspectors look out for violations like mouse droppings or torn screen doors that might allow insects into milking parlors. They make sure the flooring of barns is cleaned properly. They also periodically take milk samples to be tested for pathogens.

Before 2006, the inspection process was a tedious, but tolerable, affair for the Smiths and other raw dairy producers. Under the manual system in place, the dairy inspectors generally took a cooperative attitude with the farmers they inspected each month. So if they found that a screen door leading to the milking parlor had a tear, they might tell the farmer, so he could repair it and avoid receiving a citation. But in 2006, the department implemented an automated process. Violations were checked off on a form, and when inspectors returned to their offices, they'd enter the data into a computer.

Violations were akin to automobile traffic tickets. Different types of violations were worth varying numbers of points. Gone was the old flexibility of give-and-take where small problems could be deferred and cleaned up in time for a reinspection. Instead farmers were rated at any of three levels—level 1 being perfect, level 2 showing a few violations, and level 3 showing more serious problems, leading to an immediate fine and the necessity of reinspection within thirty days.

By the end of 2006, the Smiths had received several level 3 ratings, based on seemingly small problems like weeds around the dairy and mouse droppings too near the milking area—the kinds of things that old-time farms took for granted as part of what makes a farm. During the summer of 2006, they were fined $500. Steve called the head of the dairy division to dispute some of the findings—by February 2007 the fine had been reduced to $250. But the same day news arrived about the reduction, there were three other letters disclosing additional violations, and fines. "We couldn't get out of this reinspection cycle," recalls Steve.

Steve and Barb felt as if they were on a treadmill whose speed was increasing to such an extent they couldn't keep up.

During 2006, the Smiths began searching ever more desperately for a way off the Ag & Markets treadmill. A conversation with a local lawyer yielded an intriguing idea: The Smiths could separate their raw milk operation from the rest of the dairy, and organize it into a limited liability company, or LLC, which is a type of corporate organization that has taken hold in many states around the country over the last decade—kind of a cross between a corporation and a partnership, the two traditional forms of formal business organization. Consumers interested in a regular supply of raw milk would buy shares in the LLC and thereby become owners of the operation, entitled to the LLC's regular production.

The Smiths fell in love with the idea. They saw it affording them several benefits. Prime among these was that, as a private venture no longer selling to the general public, their raw dairy operation would be outside the constraints of the New York Department of Agriculture and Markets. The Smiths would then presumably be able to provide delivery closer to Ithaca, expanding their reach in that lucrative market. Even better, the Smiths could begin filling the demand for other dairy products—high-value products with better margins than plain milk—and provide their shareholders raw butter, cream, kefir, and yogurt. One additional bonus: no more of those debilitating inspections, with fines for highly questionable offenses.

It would seem at first glance as if the Smiths were simply extending the cow-share concept, giving it more of a corporate wrapping than conventional cow shares, which tend to be cooperative in nature. Here is how the Farm-to-Consumer Legal Defense Fund defines a cow share:

> The consumer purchases a share in a milk cow or dairy herd. The farmer and the consumer enter into a contract whereby the farmer feeds and boards the cow, and provides the labor to milk the cow and store the consumer's milk. Such contracts are legal and valid, as guaranteed by the Constitution of the United States of America. The consumer does not buy milk from the farmer. Rather, he pays the farmer for the service of keeping the cow and his labor for milking the cow and processing the milk into butter, cream, cheese, etc. However, he may directly purchase other products from the farm, such as eggs, vegetables and meat. Cow-share programs protect the farmer from liability since the cow belongs to the consumer and the consumer is drinking the milk from his own cow.[4]

From the Smiths' perspective, cow shares worked in Michigan and Ohio; why couldn't they work in New York?

Well, as it turned out, there was one important difference between New York and those other states. New York has a permit system that allows for the sale of raw milk directly from the farm. Ohio and Michigan don't have such provisions. So what the Smiths were doing was establishing a private organization that would be outside the reach of New York's agriculture officials. Would New York's regulators go along with this logic, and allow raw milk to be distributed outside their authority?

In April 2007, the Smiths took a huge step: They returned their raw milk permit to the New York Department of Agriculture and Markets.

For a few months, all was well. The Smiths confirmed to themselves that they had come upon a much better and more profitable business model. Word of the Smiths' LLC, and the availability of pickup points closer to Ithaca than the farm, encouraged consumers to buy shares—$50 for an initial investment, and then $6 per gallon, payable in advance on a quarterly basis. Before long, they had 130 shareholders, versus the 20 to 30 customers who had previously visited their farm.

Equally encouraging to them, the financial pressures of the conventional business model eased considerably. "Selling direct [via the LLC], you can get the same income with half the number of animals," Barb explained to me in their living room, made cozy by a wood-burning stove going full blast on a cold morning in January 2008. The key was being able to get $6 a gallon for milk by going direct to consumers, rather than getting a maximum of $2 a gallon (and usually much less) by selling through a processor. Plus, they were now able to sell other raw dairy products—getting $10 a pound for butter and $3 a quart for yogurt. Raw milk butter is highly prized by raw dairy consumers because the fat is thought to aid in vitamin absorption. "I can't fill demand for butter," Barb told me.

The Smiths reduced their herd from thirty cows to fourteen. That cut costs for hay and feed by 50 percent. And because shareholders were paying in advance, both for their shares and for their milk, the Smiths' cash flow improved, reducing their borrowing costs. No more $100,000 loans. And much less stress worrying about wild fluctuations in bulk milk prices from processors.

There were two other benefits, these unanticipated by the Smiths. According to Steve, "We noticed when we started selling direct that we had a lot more pride in our product as compared to dumping it into a tanker truck."

Plus, there was feedback from shareholders, and much of that was about health improvements they experienced. "One woman had been on prescription heartburn medication for seven years," said Barb. "The first week she began drinking our milk, she went off the prescription medication, and she's never looked back."

Unfortunately for the Smiths, it didn't take long for problems to crop up. In late April, just a few weeks after returning their raw milk permit to New York's Department of Agriculture and Markets, they took a booth at an Ithaca farmer's market—the booth was a convenient pickup spot for shareholders. It was also a place to promote the LLC to prospective shareholders.

But someone (the Smiths think it was an individual from Cornell, which has an agriculture school) complained to Ag & Markets. "The farmer's market manager got a call from Ag & Markets," complaining that the Smiths were violating state regulations limiting raw milk sales to direct-from-the-farm.

The farmer's market didn't care, but Ag & Markets did. Indeed, the agency gave no credence to the LLC as a private arrangement between the Smiths and their shareholders. Instead, it treated the matter as a serious violation of state dairy laws and regulations. To gather evidence to make their case that the Smiths were illegally selling raw milk and other raw dairy products, the department dispatched an undercover agent to join the Smiths' LLC and gather evidence. In June, the investigator, Dennis C. Brandow Jr., visited the Smiths' stall at the Ithaca market. In testimony he gave at an Ag & Markets hearing the following January charging the Smiths with violating state rules and regulations covering raw milk sales, he described how he had infiltrated the LLC.

As I read through the testimony, I had to remind myself several times that the case involved raw milk and not a drug bust. Brandow recounted under questioning by a New York Ag & Markets attorney his infiltration of the Meadowsweet LLC, beginning at 11 a.m. on June 23, 2007, at the Ithaca Farmer's Market.

> Q: Did you approach a booth identified as being operated by Meadowsweet Dairy, LLC?
>
> A: Yes, I did.
>
> Q: Why don't you describe how you made that identification.
>
> A: Well, there was signage stating such.
>
> Q: And was there a person who appeared to be in charge of that booth?
>
> A: Yes.
>
> Q: And did you, at some point on that date, learn that person's name?
>
> A: Yes, I did.
>
> Q: And how did you so determine that name?
>
> A: I introduced myself, and that person did as well.
>
> Q: And what name did that person give you?
>
> A: Barbara Smith.
>
> Q: Mr. Brandow, did you determine if raw milk and raw milk products were available at this booth at that time?
>
> A: Yes.
>
> Q: And did you attempt to obtain raw milk and raw milk products when you first visited this booth?
>
> A: Yes
>
> Q: Were you able to do so?
>
> A: Not at first. I engaged Mrs. Smith in conversation and she explained to me that I had to become a member of their program and I'd have to fill out a form, which I did.

A copy of the form is then entered into the record and shown to Brandow.

Q: Could you tell us what it is?

A: It's a form identifying Meadowsweet Dairy LLC, it explains them, and there's a section on the back side where you can sign, if you become a member sign and get some information.

Q: Okay. And does that appear to be a blank copy of the form that was furnished to you by Mrs. Smith on June 23rd, 2007?

A: Yes, it does.

Q: Did you subsequently sign that form?

A: Yes, I did.

Q: What did you do with the signed copy?

A: I gave it to Mrs. Smith.

Q: And you might have mentioned this, was there also a fee associated with becoming a member of Meadowsweet Dairy, LLC?

A: Yes, there was.

Q: And how much was that fee?

A: $50 fee.

Q: And did you pay it, sir?

A: Yes, I did.

Q: How did you pay it?

A: In a cash payment.

Q: Mr. Brandow, after you paid the fee and filled out the form, were you allowed to obtain raw milk and raw milk products from Meadowsweet?

A: Yes, I was.

Q: And at what point were you allowed to do that?

A: It was a bit of time later I was advised by Mrs. Smith to come back at approximately 2:30 in the afternoon. . . . I was able to obtain two gallons, glass gallons of raw milk, which I paid $10 for; two plastic quarts of yogurt; one plastic quart of cream; and one plastic quart of kefir.

Q: Regarding the milk products, not the milk that you testified to, did you furnish any money in exchange for those milk products?

A: Yes, I did.

Q: Can you elaborate on that, please?

A: I furnished a total of $20 for the total of the products . . .

Q: Once you obtained them, what did you do with them?

A: I proceeded to walk towards my vehicle, leave the farmers market.

Q: So you took these milk and milk products with you to your vehicle?

A: Yes.

Q: How much time elapsed between the time that you obtained the products, and by "products" I mean the milk and milk products, how much time elapsed between the time you obtained them and the time that you arrived at your vehicle?

A: Very short time; I'd say five minutes or less.

Q: At the time you arrived at your vehicle, did you place these containers of raw milk and raw milk products in any type of packaging?

A: Yes, I did.

Q: Can you describe what you did in that regard, please? . . .

A: I packaged four products that day, one half-gallon of milk. I put—I inserted it into a plastic bag, assigned it an FL number on the actual glass product, put it in the bag and with a twisty secure[d] it and then use[d] a little metal clip to secure it.

Q: And you just used the term "FL .4." Why don't you tell us what you mean by that.

A: That's just an identifier for myself and the food lab so they can identify the product when I bring it to the food lab . . .

There follow three more pages about the forms.

Q: Now, you mentioned that you obtained six containers of raw milk and raw milk products on June 23rd.

A: Yes.

Q: Once you brought them to your car and put them in a bag, what do you do with them at that point?

A: Then I proceeded to put them in a cooler full of ice.

Q: Why don't you describe that cooler, please . . .

There follow two more pages of description about the cooler being "a typical picnic cooler" and how much ice it contained.

Q: Did you make any stops along the way between the time that you left to get to the farmers market and [the time] you subsequently arrived in Albany?

A: No.

Q: Was the cooler out of your possession during the period of time that you obtained these raw milk and raw milk products and [until] you arrived in Albany?

A: No.

Q: Now, you mentioned that you arrived in Albany. Once you arrived here, what did you do?

A: I went right to the food lab at the state campus, and I called Dan Rice. He's the director over at the food lab, and he came over to meet me at approximately 5:40 in the afternoon.

Q: And once Mr. Rice met with you, can you tell us what happened at that point?

A: He proceeded to escort me and the product inside the building in the food lab.

Q: At some point you were inside the building with the cooler. Is that correct?

A: Yes.

Q: What did you do with the cooler once upon arriving at the food laboratory?

A: I related to Dan Rice and Cathy Ford, particularly, who started to process the materials.

Q: And what do you mean by "processing"?

A: She started to do her testing, particularly temperature control, and started to go through the—go through the bags, and I relayed the product to her . . .

There follow about a dozen more pages of testimony by Brandow, in which he describes how he obtained additional products from the Meadowsweet LLC, and brought them to the lab for testing.

I obviously wasn't the only one who had a bad taste in my mouth as I followed this discouraging episode, blow by blow. So did Gary Cox, the

Farm-to-Consumer Legal Defense Fund lawyer. As he cross-examined Brandow about the process he went through to join the Meadowsweet LLC, he suddenly switched gears:

"When you became a member of the LLC, did you tell them that you were going to be a snitch?"

The Ag & Markets lawyer, Larry Swartz, immediately objected, and the hearing officer sustained the objection.

Behind Gary's irritation was his knowledge that the undercover agent had played on Barb Smith's natural helpfulness to entrap her. Gary noted in a comment on my blog: "With Mr. Brandow's situation, he was insistent. 'I live so far away, and I only come here so very infrequently, so can't I at least have some today, PLEEEEEEEASE, because otherwise I won't be able to get any for a long time?' Barb Smith felt sorry for him and relented. We know what the consequence was of her kindness. That's the approach these undercover agents take, they're insistent."[5]

Gary also knew that these "buys" weren't simply administrative exercises. The New York Department of Agriculture and Markets used the information Brandow supplied to launch an aggressive campaign that can only be described as harassment. It stepped up its inspections of the Smiths' dairy during July and August, and at the end of August hit Meadowsweet with a fine of $1,700 for "unsanitary plant conditions": things like a torn screen, an unlabeled bottle (which contained buttermilk), a small pool of water that collected under a refrigerator condenser, and "excessive weeds" outside the barn.

Adding insult to injury, Barbara Smith was informed that if she didn't pay the fine within fifteen days, she faced a possible lawsuit to recover the penalties. She didn't pay.

Moreover, on September 7, when an inspector showed up, she answered his question as to whether it was okay to conduct an inspection with a refusal. She reasoned that since she no longer had a raw milk permit, she should no longer be subject to inspections that seemed geared toward harassment fines. On September 14, the inspector returned, this time with a supervisor, and she once again refused to allow them to conduct an inspection.

On October 3, the same inspector and supervisor showed up, and this time they had a warrant from the New York State Supreme Court in Albany County, stating to the bureaucrats: "You are hereby authorized to enter [the farm]; to inspect those premises; to take photographs; to inspect any vehicles used for the storage or transportation of milk, dairy products and food to and from the premises; to quarantine milk, dairy products or food which is adulterated or misbranded; to take samples of milk, dairy products, and food for analysis; and to seize, destroy, or denature such items which are unfit or unsafe for use."

Barbara told them she wanted to speak with her lawyer, though she says she never refused to let the two enter her property. The inspectors said that if she wasn't going to stand aside, they would file contempt charges against her, and left.

She says she wouldn't have refused the inspectors permission to conduct their search, except they didn't give her a chance. "It feels like entrapment," she adds.

Late in the afternoon on October 3, I spoke with Jessica Chittenden, the public information officer for the New York Department of Agriculture and Markets, and she sounded a conciliatory tone, saying that the department's lawyer had just made contact with the Smiths' lawyer. "We are hopeful that the Smiths will comply with the regulations," she stated.

Which regulations? "We require a permit for the sale of raw milk," Chittenden said. When I explained that the Smiths had given up their permit and weren't selling raw milk, but rather distributing it to cow-share owners, she said, "We are in the process of negotiating all that with their lawyer."

As for possible contempt charges against the Smiths, "Nothing has been decided yet," Chittenden told me.

Pete Kennedy, a lawyer for the Farm-to-Consumer Legal Defense Fund who spoke with Barbara, told me that, in his view, New York's Department of Agriculture and Markets "exceeded their authority. There is nothing in the law that says they have jurisdiction over herd-share programs."

It's tempting to view what was happening as an isolated event, or possibly an aberration based on the fact that the Smiths were attempting a radical break with past practice in New York, and with the primary milk-regulating authority in the state. That might make sense except for a few other events that were occurring at the same time. For one thing, there was the sudden rash of listeria readings turning up in the raw milk of New York raw dairy farmers, which I described in chapter 5.

Even more evidence that this wasn't an isolated event came from neighboring Pennsylvania, which has a similar raw-dairy-permit situation as New York. During the summer and fall of 2007, while New York Ag & Markets was in the midst of ever-more-aggressive inspections of the Smith farm, the Pennsylvania Department of Agriculture was mounting its own offensive against two Mennonite raw dairy farmers, Mark Nolt and Glen Wise. Like the Smiths of Meadowsweet, Nolt and Wise had given up their raw dairy permits so they could sell directly to consumers and offer them the raw butter, cream, and yogurt that were in such great demand. And also like the New York investigations of the Smiths, these cases both began with undercover infiltrations.

The details of the undercover work in Pennsylvania also came out in official proceedings—during magistrate trials of the two dairy farmers that occurred in May 2008. And the details were every bit as depressing as in the Meadowsweet case.

Several things made the dual Pennsylvania episodes especially notable. The first was that the PDA had mounted two highly orchestrated raids on Mark Nolt's dairy—the kind normally reserved for violent drug dealers or murderers—each time sending caravans of PDA, FDA, and state police officers to seize raw dairy products and cheesemaking equipment, and to haul Mark into court to be served with citations and contempt-of-court orders for refusing to appear in court for previous citations. The officers would set up a police perimeter around the hundred-acre shaded property in Newville, in south-central Pennsylvania, and its farmhouse and farm store, and the officers warned neighbors against taking videos. The shows of force led to reports the officers had come in with guns drawn. Absolutely not, an FDA official I met at a food safety conference, and who participated in one of the raids, told me in February 2008. "We did not come in with our guns drawn." He actually seemed insulted, as if it somehow excused the fact that the armed agents descended on a farm whose owner had no history of violence. At the second raid, in April 2008, a PDA official was seen leaving the farm store carrying a copy of Joel Salatin's book, *Everything I Want to Do Is Illegal,* which the farm store offered for sale. A PDA official confirmed the seizure, and the fact that the agency hadn't paid for the book, but couldn't say why the book was taken.

The second thing that made the trials notable was that the farmers, having decided for religious reasons not to hire lawyers, handled their own legal defenses. That meant they conducted their own cross-examinations of the undercover agents. Their questions led to some unexpected disclosures, which I described in blog postings about the two events. The first involved Nolt's cross-examination of Anthony Russo, a Pennsylvania Department of Agriculture microbiologist who was turned by his boss into an undercover agent to obtain evidence against Nolt.

Russo, a lanky bearded fellow who has been with the agency 21 years, had just testified about two occasions when top PDA food safety official Bill Chirdon asked—no, demanded—that Russo accompany him on an "undercover" assignment. The undercover assignment involved going to a farmer's market near the state capital of Harrisburg and purchasing raw dairy products from Mark Nolt so he could be put on trial.

Russo's first assignment came July 6, 2007, at a farmer's market in Carlisle, and went off without a hitch, as Russo purchased a half gallon of milk and a quart of kefir, as Chirdon waited outside the market in a car. Presumably Mark would have recognized Chirdon, thus possibly endangering the well-planned and highly coordinated operation.

"I asked [Mark] about the kefir, and he said there were 13 positive bacteria in it," recalled Russo. The employee took the items back to the lab and confirmed they were, indeed, raw dairy.

A week later, Chirdon made the same request of Russo. This time, Russo hesitated. "Once again, it was a busy day at work," recalled [Russo]. "He [Chirdon] asked me to go. He's my boss, so I said I would go." [Russo] purchased half a gallon of milk and some buttermilk, and brought them to his boss waiting outside the market.

"When the judge asked Mark if he had questions for Russo, Mark inquired about who drove the car and where they parked on each occasion.

Russo answered, obviously uncomfortable about having to confront the victim of his subterfuge, because he then volunteered: "I was nervous about going. I don't like doing that kind of stuff. I was hoping you weren't there because I didn't want to get any samples."

After the trial, and the guilty verdict by Judge Day, several of the Mennonite women in the audience—easily identifiable by their bonnets and traditional dresses—approached Russo and thanked him for his honesty. He seemed touched, as well he should have been. He's just a regular guy trying to do his job, avoid trouble, and eventually get a nice pension.[6]

The very next day came the trial of Glen Wise:

With Deur [the PDA lawyer] was the PDA's main witness, Joe Goetz, a food sanitarian with the agency's Bureau of Food Safety for the last two-and-a-half years, and its undercover officer of the day. Like Tony Russo yesterday, Goetz painted a picture of an employee forced into distasteful actions, except his assignment was even more questionable than that described yesterday in the Mark Nolt case.

At first, it sounded like standard practice. "I was directed by my supervisor to make a purchase of raw milk and kefir" from Glen Wise, Goetz stated. He described how he went to the Wises' Shady Acres Dairy Farm on three occasions—November 14 [2007], January 8, and March 8 [2008]—each time purchasing half a gallon of raw milk and a quart of kefir.

But when it came time for cross-examination, Glen was ready. "Did you see the sign on the refrigerator, 'Dairy products for sale to CARE members only?'" [CARE stands for the Communities' Alliance for Responsible Eco-Farming, a private purchasing organization.]

Goetz said, "Honestly, I did not pay attention to any signs."

But it got worse. "Are you a CARE member?" Wise asked.

"Yes."

"So you did sign a CARE contract?"

"Yes."

"Did you read that contract?"

"Yes."

When Deur objected that Goetz was being asked to interpret the law, the judge intervened. "What was the purpose of the contract?"

"I was asked to sign the contract by my supervisor," Goetz answered.

The judge followed up: "What did you expect that the contract provided?"

Goetz said he couldn't recall.

The point here is very important, though. The CARE membership agreement [which requires all members to pay a $20 annual membership fee] states at the start, in bold, all caps:

"ALL CARE MEMBERS MUST INITIAL AND CERTIFY, UNDER PENALTY OF PERJURY WITH THE INTENT TO BE LEGALLY BOUND TO THE FOLLOWING . . ."

There follow eleven clauses that must be initialed indicating, for example, that the member isn't aware of any medical conditions that would prevent him or her from consuming raw dairy and supports CARE's mission statement. However, the first clause in the list states: "Whereas, that HE/SHE is not acting under color of law to entrap, hurt, prosecute, or otherwise trespass and/or gather information for any agency, corporation, person or other entity to in any way negatively affect the CARE Alliance/Association, its board of directors, members or its purpose."

"Judge Duncan hadn't seen the CARE contract in advance, but she made copies of it during a recess in the proceedings.

In her ruling, Judge Duncan said that Glen's argument that the CARE contract is a private arrangement between the farmer and the consumer, and thus outside the state's raw-milk permitting requirements, "is outside the scope of this court's authority." In effect, she was leaving the matter to the Common Pleas Court, where Glen intends to appeal the single citation he was found guilty on.[7]

The trial of Mark Nolt and the surrounding publicity did nothing to dissuade PDA authorities. In September 2008, a caravan of state police and regulators descended for a third time on his farm, once again confiscating product and equipment.

In contrast with the huge frontal assault mounted against Mark Nolt in Pennsylvania, the offensive against the Smiths in New York state was more like Chinese water torture. Gradually, ever so gradually, the authorities increased the pressure on the Smiths. In early October, Ag & Markets inspectors seized several thousand dollars' worth of raw milk, yogurt, and buttermilk from Meadowsweet's coolers. The agency also ordered the Smiths to appear at an agency hearing in late October to explain their alleged violation of the Ag & Markets requirement to sell raw milk with a permit, and not sell other raw dairy products. The Smiths refused to attend that hearing, not wanting to recognize the agency's authority over Meadowsweet's activities.

The fact that the Smiths had legal assistance helped them delay some of the agency's subsequent moves, particularly the search warrants, and to take the legal offensive. Here is how I described the situation as of mid-December 2007:

Thursday, December 20, 2007 at 10:13 p.m.

On December 11, Meadowsweet and its limited liability company's 121 owners filed suit against New York Department of Agriculture and Markets officials, seeking an end to department interference with and harassment of the LLC. On December 13, NY Ag and Markets fired back, filing a second complaint against Meadowsweet to "show cause" why it shouldn't be shut down for selling raw dairy products without a permit. The complaint ignores the fact that Meadowsweet is organized as a limited liability company, with its shareholders/raw milk consumers owning the cows.

As if to further subvert the LLC arrangement, the December 13 complaint includes a "Report of Sampling and Analysis" showing inspectors made a "purchase" of Meadowsweet milk last July at a neighboring farm (and shareholder) Meadowsweet uses as a dropoff point for shareholders to pick up milk and other products. The document shows the milk was tested for pathogens and bacteria count. The document is curious, says Barbara, since the LLC doesn't "sell" milk; she suggests that an ag inspector either must have taken the milk, without authorization, or else be a member of the LLC.

Then, last week, ag inspectors arrived during the middle of a snowstorm with a warrant to oversee destruction of products seized from the first complaint filed in October . . . and by the way, wanted to get their paws on more recent dairy products the Smiths had produced. But this time the Smiths were prepared, and called the local sheriff, who encouraged the fellas to leave, since they didn't have a warrant for the new trouble they wanted to create.

So, yesterday, the inspectors showed up again. As Barbara describes it, "Today, December 19, the inspectors returned with an inspection warrant (since we had them removed by the police last week when they came without a warrant!). The new warrant says they have the right to "enter the premises on a continuing basis . . . to quarantine food that is adulterated or misbranded . . . and to seize, destroy, or denature food or food products which are unfit or unsafe for use as food."

But the Smiths had taken some precautions in advance of this latest inspection. "We were one step ahead of them and had installed locks on the doors of our processing facility," says Barbara.

That was fortunate, because there was something missing from the warrant: the authority to "use whatever force necessary" to gain access to the products, according to Gary Cox, the lawyer who is representing the Smiths as part of the Farm-to-Consumer Legal Defense Fund.

When the Smiths called Gary and read the warrant language, he advised the Smiths "to walk away" from the inspectors. That way, if they broke the locks and confiscated product, they couldn't use it as evidence.

"There was a big hullabaloo over this yesterday at Meadowsweet Farm," says Barbara. "They apparently called for reinforcements, as a state trooper appeared on the scene while we were talking to Gary. The trooper said they did have the right to use force, but Gary insisted that the law is very clear on this and they do not. . . . After the inspectors and the trooper spent about an hour consulting with each other and after many calls to Albany for marching orders, the inspectors gave it up for the second time in a week and headed home without their coveted inspection!! AWWWW!" It sure helps to have good legal advice.

I tried twice today to reach officials at the New York Department of Agriculture and Markets to get their side to this bizarre story. A spokesperson called me back early this afternoon, after my second call, and asked if she could telephone me in a couple hours, when she was back in her office and had her notes. But I never heard anything further from her.

It's clear that NY Ag and Markets could go back to a judge for a new warrant, authorizing force. Whether they will is another question.

Gary Cox says he has had some discussions with officials at the department over the last few weeks, and hopes he can get a productive dialogue going. But it seems clear that the Smiths have the bureaucrats in a dither with their limited liability company approach for distributing raw milk.

Are the ag people perhaps a little worried that the Smiths will set a precedent for other dairy farmers seeking to serve the huge New York raw milk market—out of the reach of ag restrictions on raw-milk yogurt, butter, and other such products? Maybe then we wouldn't need so many ag bureaucrats harassing raw milk dairies.

Barbara remains upbeat for the present, but very worried about the future. "This whole experience is making me SOOOO grateful for our civil liberties and SOOO nervous that we, and especially our children, may not have them in the future!"[8]

My account prompted an interesting debate among readers. One, who ran a listserve on local farming in the Rochester area, noted that she had received a concerned note from one consumer, as follows:

> As an educator, I have mixed feelings when reading the saga that Barb and Steve Smith are facing. We are only getting their point of view on this; from all I have read and know about dairy law in NY, the Smiths engaged in an illegal activity, and appear to be seeking peer support to solve the mess. We consumers can lose our access to raw milk from organic, grass-fed dairy cattle if this is pushed too far, and I am concerned it will backfire.
>
> The laws of NY allow a farmer to sell raw milk to we consumers with a permit, and the Smiths' actions may, in the end, cause Ag and Markets to eliminate the permit for all farmers.
>
> The laws of NY do not allow a company to sell raw milk. The minute the Smiths chose to distribute raw milk under a corporate liability shield (their LLC), they violated the law. The law allows a person (not a corporation) to sell raw milk.
>
> We all know the benefits of raw milk. But since it is so easily contaminated even on the best-run dairy farms, all consumers need to be protected. Thus, corporate structures, especially those that limit liability and consumer recourse, have no place in raw milk sales. I hope the position the Smiths have taken do not have unintended consequences.

Most other readers expressed dismay that this consumer seemed to be selfish. Pete's comment was typical:

> It sounds like that consumer is coming at it from a pragmatist viewpoint; her concerns chiefly being her own access to raw milk. This is selfishness, you are protecting your own access to raw milk at the expense of others who could, but don't presently have access.
>
> It is also the attitude of a slave and not a freeman. The slave is afraid of bucking the system and losing their privileges. The

freeman lives free and fights anyone who tells him otherwise. It also belies a modern attitude of avoiding pain and discomfort, we no longer have the guts for suffering and persecution that our forefathers did . . .[9]

By January 2008, the struggle between the Smiths and Ag & Markets had moved from the dairy into courtrooms and hearing rooms. At a hearing in the old Seneca County Courthouse in Waterloo, New York, a state judge refused a request by Ag & Markets to dismiss the suit, but also refused the Smiths' request for an order barring the state from interfering with its activities.

What that meant was that a January hearing at Ag & Markets headquarters in Albany would be held. It was at that hearing, presided over by a local lawyer hired by Ag & Markets, that the major issues in the case were aired more fully than any court would subsequently permit. Earlier in this chapter, I provided excerpts from the testimony of an undercover agent, Dennis Brandow, Jr., who had secretly joined the Meadowsweet LLC to obtain raw dairy products. Following his testimony, which takes about thirty pages of transcript, there is the testimony of Cathy Ford, a senior food bacteriologist for Ag & Markets. That takes another thirty-plus pages, to essentially describe how the dairy products acquired by the undercover agent were kept at the required temperature and "were intact." Interestingly, while she notes that she tested the milk for coliforms and standard plate count (total bacteria), those numbers are never revealed. Presumably, if there was anything suspicious about those readings—that they were abnormally high, for example—the Ag & Markets attorney would have asked her about them, but he didn't.

The fact that the bacteriologist presumably didn't find anything abnormal doesn't mean that the subject didn't come up. In fact, it could be said that the shit hit the fan with testimony provided by Casey McCue, the Ag & Markets chief inspector, who showed photos suggesting that during an October 11, 2007, inspection of the Smiths' milking barn, "The north wall of the milking barn is caked with manure." He added, "This manure is a source of contamination. Manure has been documented to contain *E. coli,* campylobacter, salmonella, staph-aureus. . . . Manure [is] a source of the pathogen . . . a fly, [such as] is commonly present in a milking stable, could easily land on this manure, and through its normal digestive process of regurgitating on its food, could suck the fluid back up from this manure, which is a source of contamination, and then fly over and land on milking equipment, and further even land on the cow's udder just prior to [its] being milked."

There was never any evidence presented that Meadowsweet's milk was contaminated. In later cross-examination, Gary Cox established that no members of the LLC, many of whom had visited the farm, had ever complained about conditions at the farm. Cox even threw this question to McCue to suggest that manure is ever-present on dairy farms:

> Q: What if they [the Smiths] tracked manure, what if their
>   boots tracked manure into the milking stable; would that
>   be a violation?
> A: No, it would not.

But the damage had been done. Manure had been mentioned in the same breath as assorted pathogens and milking equipment.

Gary Cox saw his mission in the hearing as not to argue about manure— after all, not only had no one become ill, but no pathogens had been uncovered in Meadowsweet's milk—but rather to make the case that, not only was the Meadowsweet LLC not the "sham" it was labeled by the Ag & Markets lawyer, but that it was serving its shareholders.

> There's absolutely no evidence that this LLC is a sham. It's formed,
> as [Barb Smith] testified, for the purpose of making raw milk and
> raw dairy product [available] to its members. There is nothing ille-
> gal in New York law for that to happen. So when I say we need to
> think outside the box, we need to think of an LLC that's not in the
> business of making money. It's not in the business of selling wid-
> gets or making widgets and putting those widgets into the stream
> of interstate commerce. This LLC was created to make raw milk and
> raw dairy products available only to its members.
>
> Until the law changes, in New York, this is not an illegal activity.
> It's not regulated by Ag and Markets; it's not subject to the per-
> mitting and licensing requirements; it doesn't involve any sales to
> consumers; and it's not adversely impacting or injuring the public's
> health safety or welfare.
>
> This is a group of people who have decided amongst themselves,
> "We're opting out of the government's sanctioned industrial dairy

system. We're going to produce our own milk and our own dairy products and we're going to consume them. It's our own free choice."

NY Ag & Markets was quick to let Gary Cox and the Smiths know that it wasn't about to bend in the least. In February, it filed suit in state court to have the Smiths jailed for contempt of court for their alleged failure to abide by the search warrants of December. Apparently the state of New York wasn't about to be outdone by neighboring Pennsylvania in its willingness to stand up and show toughness against raw dairy farmers.

Ultimately, in a late-March court session, a state judge refused to declare the Smiths in contempt, reasoning that the court suit they had filed in December would help resolve the whole issue. If the Smiths were successful, and the Meadowsweet LLC was seen to be outside the Ag & Markets purview, then the contempt request would be moot.

So the Smiths were protected, at least temporarily, until their court suit was decided.

CHAPTER ELEVEN

Nine Words Ignite a Raw Milk Battle, California-Style

On a Wednesday evening, October 19, 2007, I received a telephone call from Mark McAfee, the owner of Organic Pastures Dairy Co. in Fresno, California. He said he had some "important news" that he wanted to share with me.

A bit of seemingly routine dairy legislation had recently passed the California legislature and just been signed into law. It was known as AB 1735, and it made some adjustments to the complex regulations surrounding pasteurized milk. But within that legislation were nine words inserted by the California Department of Food and Agriculture, supposedly to align California's milk law with FDA guidelines, Mark explained.

Those nine words stipulated that raw milk "shall contain not more than . . . 10 coliform bacteria per milliliter."[1]

At the time I didn't know what McAfee was talking about, what coliforms even were, but I did know that, though he had strong opinions on lots of things, Mark didn't use the word *important* very often. Little could I have imagined those nine legislative words would ignite a food storm in the largest state's politics for more than a year, until finally it was resolved, at least temporarily, by Governor Arnold Schwarzenegger.

It would be many months before I understood that the planning and plotting to make life more difficult for Organic Pastures—which Stephen Beam of the CDFA started almost immediately after the quarantining of the Organic Pastures dairy in September 2006 (described in chapter 2)—had come to fruition. The last major component of the Golden State's campaign against raw milk was just being revealed and about to burst into public view.

Whereas the battle over Meadowsweet Dairy LLC, described in the previous chapter, was fought outside of public view, in hearing rooms and on lonely farm roads, the battle over raw milk in California was fought loudly, boisterously, in full public view. While there was definitely a good deal of behind-the-scenes politicking, much of California's raw milk drama played out the way one might expect in California—complete with colorful characters and weird turns of events.

I had gotten to know McAfee pretty well over the previous year, since his dustup with the CDFA and other regulatory agencies in connection with the suspected contamination of his milk with *E. coli* O157:H7 and the illnesses of six children, including Chris Martin, in September 2006 (described in chapters 2 and 9) allegedly caused by raw milk. There had been the back-and-forth comments on my blog with Mary McGonigle-Martin, described in chapter 9, in which he challenged her claim that Chris had become ill from his milk. There was the run-in with the US Food and Drug Administration described in chapter 5 over a finding of listeria in his cream.

Mark McAfee had by this time become a central figure in the new generation of raw milk battles being fought around the country. His Organic Pastures Dairy Co. was by far the largest raw dairy in the country, having grown, by his own estimates, to serving thirty-five to forty thousand customers each day via more than three hundred retail outlets, including dozens of Whole Foods groceries. That accomplishment was thanks in significant measure to the fact that California is one of only a few states that allow retail sales of raw milk (apart from on-farm direct sales), and the only one in the country that allows the retail sale of such raw dairy products as cream, butter, and kefir. It's also due to McAfee's aggressive and entrepreneurial approach to the marketplace since he transformed his four-hundred-acre Fresno-area farm into a raw dairy back in 1999.

One thing I had discovered early on about McAfee: He is extremely open and verbose, sometimes to such an extreme that he would tell me things I thought he'd be better off keeping to himself. For example, just that fall he had been telling me about his negotiations with a New York venture capital outfit that he said was potentially interested in investing many millions to help Organic Pastures upgrade its facilities, based on the VC's view of raw milk as a "disruptive" business. I had to laugh when Mark told me that—yes, raw milk was about as disruptive as you could get.

As a journalist who had been involved in writing extensively about venture capital and entrepreneurship for twenty years, I knew that business owners usually didn't discuss their negotiations with venture capitalists until the deals were concluded. The VCs generally preferred privacy until all the i's were dotted and t's crossed, and such negotiations could take many months. Yet McAfee had actually allowed me to write about his negotiations on my blog.[2]

I also learned he was a lightning rod, a man who not only didn't duck controversy but actually seemed to seek it out. After the September 2006 shutdown of his dairy, McAfee had demanded $100,000 in compensation from the CDFA to reimburse the losses associated with being shut down, arguing that he was entitled since no pathogens had been found in his milk. He wound up settling for $11,000—according to the written settlement agreement, because both parties wished to "avoid the uncertainty, adverse publicity, and discomfort of a continued conflict concerning the propriety and value of the loss suffered by OP."

While he claimed the settlement exonerated his dairy in the 2006 illnesses, the CDFA clearly didn't intend it as such. In fact, the department has frequently compensated producers for losses following a quarantine order for disease control—though most often quarantines are enacted to control the spread of animal diseases that threaten the livestock population (for example, foreign animal diseases), and not shutdowns intended to protect consumers from possibly contaminated products, which was the stated concern in the 2006 OP case.

In conversations with McAfee, I gradually learned about what drew him into the raw milk business and how, in retrospect, it was only natural that he would wind up there. He was the fourth generation of McAfee to run the four-hundred-acre farm in California's vast Central Valley, which had grown almonds, alfalfa, and apples, among other crops, over the years.

Before devoting himself full-time to the farm, though, he had spent fourteen years as a paramedic. He "retired" in 1997 to farm apples full-time. "I was at the top of my game" as a paramedic, he told me. "I was making good money, but I was tired of not sleeping nights."

He had gotten a taste of the downs of farm-life economics when, in 1995, the American market for apples was rocked by the economic buzzsaw known as China. That nation's big push into the apple market had driven down prices worldwide. McAfee continued farming apples, but was on the lookout for ways to diversify.

In 1999, he thought he'd found the answer: organic (pasteurized) milk. The organic movement was picking up speed, and dairy processors desperately needed organic product to meet rising consumer demand. They would pay premiums of 20 to 50 percent over the prices of conventional milk to farmers who fed their cattle pasture or grains certified as organic under federal regulations. McAfee decided that Organic Pastures would become "the undairy."

He obtained a contract from a major processor, but then did something few farmers did in those days—he built a Web site. The site attracted the attention of several Hollywood types, including Janet Sheen, the wife of actor Martin Sheen. These folks wanted unpasteurized milk because, like many health food devotees, they were convinced of raw milk's nutritional superiority. What's more, they were motivated most immediately by their desire to replace their previous supplier of raw milk, Alta Dena, which was just ending its sales of Stueve's Natural, a line of unpasteurized milk that had kept raw milk drinkers satisfied since the 1940s. Indeed, until a federal court ordered the FDA to implement a ban on interstate sales of raw milk in 1987, Stueve's Natural had been available in health food stores in several states besides California.

Alta Dena had grown from a few dozen cows in the 1940s to some eight thousand by the 1980s, and its raw milk production was way beyond anything around today. The cows were raised and milked just as on many current conventional dairies—crowded into feedlot-style conditions and grain-fed (in contrast with today, when nearly all raw dairies tout their pasture-based feeding for nutritionally superior milk). By the 1970s and 1980s, Alta Dena's production methods were becoming a regular source of controversy.

According to its backers, the milk didn't make people sick. "For over 40 years, Alta Dena proved that safe and healthy raw dairy products could be produced and distributed on a large scale with literally no proven cases caused by their products," states Ron Schmid, author of *The Untold Story of Milk*, in a report on the site of the Weston A. Price Foundation.[3]

According to the Schmid report, California public health officials launched a campaign, beginning in the 1960s and continuing on and off through the 1980s, to suggest that the huge dairy's milk was contaminated with various pathogens. In 1978, when Alta Dena sought legislative action to require public health officials to treat raw milk like other foods, more than fifty thousand letters in support of raw milk were sent to the governor's office.[4]

A separate report, though, by an anti-raw-milk organization, maintains that substantial numbers of Californians had become ill from salmonella, and that between 1971 and 1974, thirty-two of the seventy-nine people who became ill from salmonella were made sick by Alta Dena raw milk. It was no different in the 1980s, argued the analysis: "Alta Dena financed an independent study by the UCLA School of Public Health to determine if CRM was actually a problem. Epidemiologists at UCLA estimated that more than one-third of reported *S. dublin* infections in California from 1980–83 were attributable to raw milk consumption. It appeared that the incidence of infection was 8 to 35 per 100,000."[5]

A retrospective look at raw milk's dangers to California consumers by the California Department of Food and Agriculture, filed in early 2009 in connection with eventual legal action growing out of AB 1735, made this statement: "Since 1976, in California alone, there have been ten documented disease outbreaks associated with raw milk. One of these outbreaks resulted in a death, and another in kidney failure." So over a period of thirty-three years, the worst that an agency seeking to paint raw milk in the worst light could come up with was that raw milk consumption had resulted in one death and one case of kidney failure.[6]

Part of the problem facing Alta Dena, though, was that health inspectors were finding evidence of pathogens, especially salmonella, in the dairy's milk. Even though it was unclear how many people became ill, the news articles generated by the discoveries ate into the dairy's credibility, and business, not to mention that they created mounting legal bills. Such relentless government pressure on a particular supplier takes its toll. Yes, the business can fight back with court suits and lobbying efforts, but in the final analysis the government has more money and other resources at its disposal than pretty much any business. Eventually, in 1999, Alta Dena concluded it was fighting a losing battle against the government, and it discontinued sales of Stueve's Natural.[7]

It was against this backdrop—a backdrop that would have scared off many sensible businesspeople—that McAfee decided to enter the raw milk business shortly after Alta Dena pulled Stueve's. As he recalls it, the Hollywood types "started filling up their milk bottles" at his dairy. They didn't care about paying $12 a gallon for milk. They sent their friends. "After a couple weeks, it was ridiculous" how much milk he was selling, and how much money he was making—more than six times the price he was receiving from the processor.

Along with Janet Sheen was a California food eccentric by the name of Aajonus Vonderplanitz, who had fought hard against California health officials during the 1980s and 1990s battles over Stueve's. I use the term *eccentric* because he espouses an unusual approach to diet: consumption of an all-raw diet—not only raw milk, but raw eggs and vegetables, even raw chicken and beef. It's an approach that even the strongest raw milk supporters sometimes find distasteful—they may want their milk raw, but they like their beef and chicken cooked through.

Sheen, Vonderplanitz, and others "sat me down and told me the history of raw milk in California," McAfee recalls. When they explained the perceived health benefits of raw milk, "I understood it immediately. It made perfect sense that unpasteurized milk would help people's immunity." A number of these raw milk supporters wrote out checks and handed over cash to McAfee in the form of an informal investment in his raw milk business.

So where other business owners might have seen potential trouble in how Alta Dena was dragged down over the years, McAfee saw opportunity. Sanitation practices had improved significantly, and pasture feeding of cows seemed to lower the risks of pathogen contamination even further over conventional feedlot approaches. "I went to Whole Foods and they put it right on their shelves," he remembers. From there, it was practically a straight line up to nearly $5 million in sales by late 2006, as demand for unpasteurized milk skyrocketed.

One other factor that may have convinced McAfee he could weather regulatory storms is that he grew up in a family environment where political protest was front and center. His father, Rodger McAfee, was a serious political activist who had numerous run-ins with the government. At one point in the early 1960s, Rodger flew to Cuba in defiance of US rules and was jailed for a few weeks. Then, in 1970, he pledged the Fresno farm as collateral to post the $100,000 bail for Angela Davis, a supporter of the radical Black Panthers, who was jailed in connection with the murder of a California judge, and eventually found not guilty in a high-profile trial in 1972. (Rodger died in an auto accident in 2006.)

At heart, though, Rodger was a farmer. "We didn't have much growing up," recalls Mark. "We didn't grow up poor, but rather simple. I grew up with the idea of owning dirt. It was the only thing we owned. My father always said if you own land, you'll never be poor."

McAfee doesn't deny that his own political alienation has emerged via the raw milk revolution, but adds that, from a political perspective, "I'm far more dangerous than my father was. He had a cause for a while, and then let it go. I've got a cause in a chokehold and won't let go."

McAfee is a square-jawed, solidly built man who has shown repeatedly that he won't easily let go of what he considers right. In 2003 and 2004, there was a run-in with the FDA over his sales of raw dairy products via his Web site to out-of-state customers, who tend to live in states where raw milk is outlawed. Selling raw milk across state lines is a violation of a prohibition on interstate sales of raw milk instituted by the FDA in 1987 (discussed in the next chapter). McAfee says the prohibition applied only to milk for human consumption, so he decided to label his milk as "for pets only." The FDA didn't challenge him, at least initially.

Tough guy that he is, McAfee made another enemy along the way: his chief competitor, Claravale Farm, and its owner Ron Garthwaite. Garthwaite is the exact opposite of McAfee. Where McAfee is outspoken, Garthwaite is quiet. Where McAfee is more marketer than farmer, Garthwaite is more farmer than marketer. And where McAfee tends to see conspiracies around every corner, Garthwaite is more trusting of authority.

He and his wife, Collette Cassidy, had acquired Claravale in 1997 as a functioning dairy that had been in business since the 1920s. Their sales had grown more slowly than those of Organic Pastures, and at about $1 million annually, were about 20 percent those of Organic Pastures.

While McAfee and Garthwaite were the only two licensed sellers of raw milk in California, and seemingly had enough business to keep each of their operations running at full capacity, their differences led to some bad blood that kept them on separate paths. There had been a serious collision between the two when Mark was ramping up to expand Organic Pastures' retail operation.

Back in 2001, Organic Pastures lured a key distributor, covering the Los Angeles area, away from Claravale, in what Garthwaite says was a less-than-forthright way. "From one day to the next, we lost our Los Angeles market," he told me. "We had to send half our cows to slaughter," and the dairy just barely avoided folding.

McAfee denies he did anything underhanded, contending the distributor was eager to work for Organic Pastures because Claravale wasn't predictable enough in its milk production. While Claravale recovered, amid the growing demand for raw milk, the two men avoided each other.

Despite the irritation McAfee caused to regulators and his chief competitor, he seemed unstoppable. But late on a Friday afternoon, September 21, 2006, it all seemed to come to a crashing halt when two agents from California's Department of Food and Agriculture stopped at his dairy's nondescript single-story main office to deliver two notices: a recall order and quarantine notice. They suspected milk from Organic Pastures contained the pathogen *E. coli* O157:H7, and said that McAfee would have to recall his dairy products from two hundred retail outlets around the state, as well as halting all shipments of goods and animals to and from the dairy.

The worst part of the agents' visit, though, was their explanation for why they were suspicious: State public health authorities had learned of at least four children around the state who had become ill from the same pathogen (the number would eventually grow to six), and all appeared to have consumed an Organic Pastures product. "They told me some might die," McAfee recalls. "I was having a stroke."

Clarity returned quickly, though, and after setting in motion a recall and quarantine, McAfee set about trying to find the sick children. Under privacy laws, public health officials can't release that information, but McAfee used his paramedic experience and some old contacts to track the kids, and two days later he was in the hospital rooms of the two most seriously ill children—seven-year-old Chris Martin and ten-year-old Lauren Herzog—at Loma Linda University Medical Center, near Los Angeles.

He quickly concluded that the situation wasn't quite as grave as the CDFA agents had led him to believe. "I expected these kids to be there with the priest by the bed," McAfee recalls. Apparently they had been extremely ill some days earlier, to the extent they had been on kidney dialysis machines, but now seemed well on the road to recovery.

The key issue for McAfee then turned to what had made the children sick. He says the parents told him that, in addition to consuming raw milk, the children had eaten fresh spinach. The nation at that time was in the midst of a scare over *E. coli* O157:H7 in packaged spinach, which would sicken two hundred people, and kill three (described in chapter 8).

"It was one of those things where the reality was a lot different than what I had been told," says McAfee.

As I described in chapter 1, Mark came through the confrontation with his business intact. And, as mentioned in chapter 9, via his exchanges with Mary McGonigle-Martin, the question of what had actually made the children sick was a subject of considerable debate.

So while McAfee immediately resumed selling his raw dairy products after the quarantine was lifted in late September 2006, the CDFA's chief dairy official, Stephen Beam, began drafting the coliform standard that would come to be known as AB 1735 (as I recounted from his deposition testimony in chapter 2). When I met him in person at a dairy regulator conference in April 2009, Beam confirmed again that the illnesses attributed to Organic Pastures had driven him to action. "I thought we had a safety problem that we needed to solve," he said. The ten-coliform-per-milliliter standard, in his estimation, would serve as an indicator of whether manure that could carry the *E. coli* O157:H7 pathogen had potentially contaminated the milk.

So what was wrong with AB 1735? McAfee argued that keeping the coliform count down so low would have the effect of eliminating good bacteria as well, which are helpful in building our immune systems.

No, AB 1735 had nothing to do with milk safety, argued McAfee in our conversation of October 19. "It's payback time," he told me. The fact that he hadn't been invited to testify or otherwise comment on the proposed change represented a deliberate oversight.

"It was a Trojan horse," he said of the legislation. "We've got a tiger by the tail."

What is problematic about keeping coliform counts under ten per milliliter? Coliform readings generally vary in a wider range than the one to ten required by AB 1735. "We could have from two to hundreds," McAfee said. "Sometimes it's two, sometimes it's eight, sometimes it's twelve, twenty-four, and so on up the line." Moreover, coliforms are among the most beneficial of bacteria in milk, he explained—a good part of the reason many people want their milk unpasteurized. "California has never tested for coliforms." He ventured that up to three-quarters of Organic Pastures' milk would not pass.

McAfee's explanation and numerical estimates about coliform represented just the first launch in a dizzying propaganda battle that would ensue about a subject most people had never heard of: coliforms.

In the publicity that followed McAfee's divulgence of the import of AB 1735, the CDFA seemed in its initial public statements to both disagree and agree with him about the difficulties raw dairy producers would have complying with it. In a press release, the agency said that, based on measurements it had taken of coliforms at the two California raw dairies, as part of its overall inspections, Organic Pastures, and the smaller producer, Claravale Farms, should be able to pass 75 percent of the time. There was no acknowledgment that not too many businesses can afford to have 25 percent of their production regularly rendered unacceptable.[8]

But in a separate Q&A seeking to justify the change, CDFA said that the great majority of conventional dairies could probably pass the test only 20 to 25 percent of the time, indicating that 75 to 80 percent of all milk that goes to processors would register coliform readings in excess of 10 coliforms/milliliter before pasteurization.[9]

Beyond the numbers, those behind AB 1735 argued that the coliform count was indicative of a milk's overall cleanliness, since coliforms come primarily from fecal matter. Thus, a high coliform count, in their estimation, suggested the milk had somehow been in contact with manure, and thus was likelier than low-coliform milk to contain pathogens. In other words, coliform readings could be seen as predictive of the likelihood of pathogens like *E. coli* O157:H7, campylobacter, and salmonella.

Not true at all, argued McAfee and others who spoke out against AB 1735. Milk could come out of a cow with one or two coliforms per milliliter, and then multiply rapidly as the milk made its way to the bulk tank and then through the bottling process. By providing that the coliform measurements in California be made after bottling, AB 1735 was different from similar coliform provisions in other states, which stipulated that the measurement could be made in the bulk tank, before the agitation of bottling occurs.

McAfee's solution when we spoke that Wednesday evening in October was to somehow "return" the legislation for reconsideration. However, having majored in political science in college, I knew that, once a piece of legislation has been signed into law, it is very difficult to overturn it, at least until it has a chance to be implemented for some period of time, and is found to be problematic.

McAfee didn't care what I thought, and immediately embarked on a campaign to overturn AB 1735. One quick indication that this wasn't just Mark McAfee, the maverick, battling the regulators, occurred when Ron Garthwaite, the owner of Claravale, patched up his long-term dispute with McAfee and joined him in opposition to AB 1735.

In a classic case of "my enemy's enemy is my friend," Garthwaite—the quiet, introverted farmer—went public with his outrage over AB 1735. In early November 2007 I posted this account of Garthwaite's transformation on my blog:

> It's not been an easy year for Ronald Garthwaite, the owner of Claravale Farm, California's "other" producer of raw milk, with about 50 cows and 5 percent of the market after Organic Pastures.
>
> Last June, he had to sell his Santa Cruz County farm because he was unable to get local officials to approve the permits he needed to continue in operation. He moved to San Benito County and quickly obtained all the permits and seemed to finally have found a new and welcoming home, with his partner, Collette Cassidy.
>
> As part of the move, he built a new dairy facility—investing on the order of $1 million. Then came the late-October surprise of AB 1735, the legislation that sets a 10-coliform-per-milliliter limit on raw milk.

What's made AB 1735 especially shocking to Ronald is that he was submitting plans and having inspections by the California Department of Food and Agriculture during recent months. "Had they informed us of this new regulation we could have made changes to the facilities in order to have a better chance of meeting the new regulation," he says in an email he just sent to his customers. "Or we may have decided not to build at all. Or we may have decided to construct it to produce products other than raw milk.

"The fact that they went ahead and let us sell our house and go into significant debt to build a facility that they knew they were going to shut down within a couple months of its completion indicates that they are anything but helpful. Not only do they appear to want our dairy to fail, but they seem to want to totally destroy us personally."

The new requirement seems to have hit Ronald even harder than Mark McAfee, since Ronald says he trusted the CDFA. "For many years now we have been telling our customers that there is no conspiracy within the CDFA to eliminate raw milk; that the state was actually very supportive of the product. We were dead wrong. I'm sorry for having misled you.

"They are simply much more devious, two-faced, and sinister than I could ever have imagined. The reasons that they state for incorporating this new regulation are so transparently false, and the highly secretive method of its introduction so obviously inappropriate, that I think that there can be no doubt that the CDFA is on a mission to hobble the raw milk industry in California."

He accuses the CDFA of having spread the rumor that Claravale Farm is in favor of the law. "In some weird-bureaucratic-alien-space logic they say that since we didn't say anything against it we must be for it. Of course we didn't say anything against it because we, like everyone else, knew nothing about it. We didn't inform them that we were against it because they never informed us of its existence. Let me be clear: we are not in favor of this law."

Like Mark McAfee, he argues that the coliform requirement has been completely misrepresented by the CDFA. "The coliform bacteria in our milk do not come from manure contamination," Ronald writes.

"I am so sick and tired of the CDFA telling people that our milk is contaminated with feces. It is not true. Our milk is not contaminated with feces.

"They seem to think that if they say it enough people will believe it. It doesn't matter how many times they say it, it is not true. I repeat: Our milk is not contaminated with feces. The fact that the milk in our bulk tank meets the coliform limits for sterilized (i.e., pasteurized) milk demonstrates this fact absolutely and conclusively. At Claravale farm we have been producing high-quality, clean, safe, raw milk for over 80 years. We know how to milk cows. I would take exception to the CDFA's statement that most coliform bacteria come from feces, but whether they do or not, it is an irrelevant, inflammatory statement."

He adds, "The reason why it is so important to the CDFA that you think that there is cow manure in our milk is that they are trying to play off of the recent hysteria over produce and beef illnesses due to pathenogenic coliform. They are trying to create a raw milk hysteria that will get people to support their bill. In other words, they think you're not very smart."

He takes issue with the CDFA contention that the 10-coliform-per-milliliter standard is being applied to other states like Nevada, Arizona, Utah, Idaho, and Washington, since "There are no raw milk industries in these states."

And he accuses the CDFA of "a classic and blatantly obvious lie of omission" for failing in its fact sheet to point out that Connecticut, Idaho, and New Mexico allow 50-coliform-per-milliliter and Missouri allows 100 per milliliter.

And like Mark, he points out that the difficulty in meeting the new standard comes in the CDFA's intention to measure coliform after the milk is bottled, rather than when it is in the milk tank. "Coliform contamination is a surface area phenomenon. No surface is 100% cleanable. The more surface area the milk is required to come in contact with, the more coliform will be in the final product."

He argues that even non-raw-milk consumers should be concerned. "This is only one additional step in the state's campaign to pasteurize or sterilize everything."

His advice to Californians: "If you want to continue to be able to get Claravale milk or any raw milk in California, you need to fight this law with everything you have."[10]

Shortly after Garthwaite's public revelations, he and McAfee completely healed their old rift when they teamed up and hired a former-legislator-turned-lobbyist for $10,000 a month to try to overturn AB 1735.

One of the biggest obstacles facing the two dairies in gaining clarity was another individual with a flair for the dramatic—Nicole Parra, the chairperson of the California Assembly's Agriculture Committee. In the days that followed media revelations about the implications of AB 1735, Parra's office was deluged by phone calls and e-mails from raw milk drinkers protesting the legislation that had originated in her committee.

She quickly sent out a response that said:

> Unfortunately, recent information falsely asserts that AB 1735 will ban raw milk sales in the State of California. You will be pleased to learn that, contrary to misconceptions, AB 1735 does not ban the sale of raw milk in California.
>
> AB 1735 requires a coliform count of less than 10 per milliliter for raw fluid milk intended for direct human consumption. This standard has been implemented in a number of other states, and as their experience suggests, the standard set by AB 1735 will not affect the availability of raw milk in California.... Passing AB 1735 was a way for the Legislature to fulfill our responsibility to help protect the public health, while acknowledging the needs of those who produce and drink raw milk.[11]

The whole matter became even more contentious as 2007 drew to a close and a new year began. For one thing, the families of the two children—Chris Martin and Lauren Herzog—who became most seriously ill in September 2006 (attributed by the state to *E. coli* O157:H7–contaminated raw milk)—filed suit against Organic Pastures (described at greater length in chapters 2 and 9).[12,13]

Another development was that, during the last week of December, the Farm-to-Consumer Legal Defense Fund filed suit against the CDFA on behalf of Organic Pastures and Claravale. It argued that the state had violated several important constitutional protections afforded the dairies, including due process and equal protection under the law.[14]

The dairies' suit only seemed to intensify government resolve, and this time from "the Governator." During the first week of January, Nicole Parra's justification for AB 1735 was followed up by a much more inflammatory endorsement—from Governor Arnold Schwarzenegger. His office began sending out responses to individuals who had written him, and several forwarded the e-mails to me. He harked back to the illnesses of September 2006 to justify his backing of AB 1735—something not even CDFA had done (at least not openly) to justify the legislation.

"Raw milk has been known to be a source of foodborne illness for decades," the letter declared. "For example, in September 2006, the California Department of Public Health linked six cases of infection with the deadly *E. coli* O157:H7 to the consumption of raw milk. The median age of the victims was 8 years old. In recent years, illness outbreaks have been attributed to raw milk consumption in several states. In fact, raw milk sold for direct human consumption is illegal in all or part of 42 states."

I had to keep reminding myself this was California—the land of fantasy and fairy tales—because by late January 2008, things got even stranger on the government side as Nicole Parra did an about-face. Mark McAfee had managed to meet with her and convince her that an injustice had been done—enough of an injustice that she introduced a new piece of legislation, AB 1604, to repeal AB 1735. McAfee rallied his customers via e-mails and his Web site, and a few hundred people—McAfee says five hundred—traveled to Sacramento and jammed a hearing room in the California Assembly to hear individuals in favor testify for the repeal.

After negotiating with other committee members, Parra revised AB 1604 to repeal AB 1735 for six months, at which time a new coliform standard would be implemented, likely fifty coliforms per milliliter.[15]

At the committee hearing, Assemblywoman Parra gave an emotional speech in which she explained her about-face, and in the process castigated the CDFA. "I'm here to fix a wrong," she declared. Of the CDFA, she asked, "How hard would it have been to phone them [Organic Pastures and Claravale] and bring them into the process?"

She noted that she had never drunk raw milk. "I'm not here to say 10 coliforms per milliliter is good or bad. . . . We never got the opportunity to ask the questions," because the legislation was packaged as "a committee bill" that was simply voted on without hearings, based on the CDFA's endorsement. She added, "I want to learn more about raw milk . . . I want to drink a glass." (Her full speech is captured on a YouTube video.)[16]

Afterward, Mark McAfee was beaming. He had led a group of raw milk consumers and experts to testify on behalf of raw milk. "I'm so proud of her," he said of Nicole Parra. "I feel like such a good American. . . . This was the highlight of perhaps my adult life." (His comments are also on a YouTube video.)[17]

Barely a week later, though, the euphoria had dissipated. After passing the Agriculture Committee, AB 1604 mysteriously stalled in the Appropriations Committee, where it also needed approval (standard procedure). Apparently the CDFA had some important supporters on the committee. Upon learning of the problems, Nicole Parra pulled the legislation rather than face a possibly humiliating defeat.

Almost unnoticed in all the tumult, AB 1735 had become law on January 1, so the CDFA was free to begin enforcing it. And enforce it the CDFA did.

By late February, McAfee's worst predictions were coming true. Under a fail-three-of-five-tests-and-you're-out system (out in the sense that you receive a "de-grade" and can't sell in that product category until you pass a test), Organic Pastures quickly failed three tests on its cream and was forced to pull it off the market. The cost: more than $10,000 a week in lost revenues. More ominously, Organic Pastures failed two of the first four tests on the dairy's big enchilada, raw milk, accounting for the majority of sales.

"If I fail a third test for my raw/whole milk, I will have to cease selling raw/ whole milk and my business will collapse," McAfee stated in an affidavit to a state judge in late February.[18]

Meanwhile, the Farm-to-Consumer Legal Defense Fund was seeking to force immediate judicial action on its December suit by seeking a temporary restraining order to suspend enforcement of AB 1735. The FTCLDF was convinced that only a preliminary injunction, preventing the CDFA from enforcing AB 1735, would prevent the agency from cutting off California's flow of raw milk to an estimated forty thousand or so regular consumers.

Even as things moved into the serious confines of a courtroom, the outside atmosphere turned more bizarre. For one thing, a simmering conflict within the raw milk movement was becoming increasingly public, and acrimonious. It turned out that Aajonus Vonderplanitz, the longtime activist on behalf of raw milk in California, and early supporter of Organic Pastures' entry into the raw milk business, didn't approve of the Farm-to-Consumer Legal Defense Fund's legal strategy. So much so that he advocated a separate suit, a class-action suit based on the argument that cutting off raw milk to California citizens would damage the health of many individuals. He figured that deposing thousands of California raw milk drinkers would turn the situation into the spectacle it needed to become.[19]

Even though some in the raw milk movement ridiculed his eccentric dietary approach, the reality was that Vonderplanitz was the dean of the raw milk movement. He had directly challenged public health officials who went after Alta Dena in the 1980s and 1990s, putting together elaborate printed packages highlighting research that suggested raw milk was both safe and nutritious. As recently as the summer of 2007, he had spent several weeks in Washington personally lobbying legislators to ease restrictions on raw milk—lobbying that eventually led to proposals by Representative Ron Paul to lift a federal ban on interstate shipments of raw milk, which had been in place since 1987.[20]

At this point, though, his nutritional counseling kept him on the road more than half the time, conducting seminars and workshops on the benefits of a raw food diet. When I first spoke to Vonderplanitz the previous December, he had called me from Thailand. It wasn't clear he had the necessary bandwidth to launch a separate suit.

In mid-March, a state judge heard the Organic Pastures/Claravale case. It was argued by Gary Cox, the intense Ohio lawyer who, as a private attorney, had won the Ohio herd-share case on behalf of Carol Schmitmeyer (described in chapter 4). Only now he was working on behalf of the Farm-to-Consumer Legal Defense Fund.

Cox presented evidence not only that the dairies would suffer significant losses, but that the need for a coliform standard was based on faulty science. For example, Ted Beals, the Michigan pathologist who had overseen the study of lactose intolerance I described in chapter 7, stated in an affidavit, "Although traditionally, coliforms may be an indicator of environmental contamination, the presence of coliforms is not an indicator of the presence of pathogens."

Beals noted that "subtle increases in temperature can cause enormous increases in coliform count in a milliliter of milk over time. For example, a package of raw milk that is shipped under appropriate conditions may be placed on a grocery store shelf that is not properly refrigerated, causing an increase in the number of coliforms present over time. In addition, several packages of raw milk may be so closely packed together on a shelf in a grocery store that the inside packages of raw milk are not adequately refrigerated, another cause of increased coliforms present over time."

His conclusion: "A more proper standard would be the absence of pathogens in the bulk tank where the raw milk is stored prior to packaging."[21]

The state's lawyers essentially countered that AB 1735 wasn't nearly as ominous as portrayed. To the argument that Organic Pastures was close to being driven out of business, the state argued that the company had been reinstated to sell cream, and even when it was forced out of the cream market, "it could use the restricted raw cream to make its butter." Moreover, the state also said that during the cream shutdown, "The Department placed no restriction on Organic Pastures' sale of raw skim milk, raw whole milk, butter or cheese."

From a larger perspective, the state argued that California's coliform standard wasn't out of line. It noted that out of thirteen states, California included, allowing retail sales of raw milk (separate from direct on-farm sales to consumers), seven have the same ten-coliform-per-milliliter standard. "Plaintiffs claim that there is no way for them to meet the new standard, but this is belied by the experience of producers in other states, which have been able to meet the 10 milliliter coliform standard and stay in business."

And just to add an exclamation point to its argument, the state pointed to warnings about raw milk from the American Academy of Pediatrics and the FDA. "Even the state of Oregon, which does allow the sale of raw milk, issued a warning about the dangers of raw milk," it stated.[22]

I was expecting the judge to accept the state's arguments and the warnings about the dangers of raw milk. But much to my surprise, after hearing the arguments, the judge indicated he was swayed by the financial dangers to Organic Pastures and Claravale, and issued a temporary restraining order blocking implementation of AB 1735. Though the order really was only temporary—until a hearing on a temporary injunction could be heard a couple of months later—it was perceived as a huge victory by Mark McAfee and raw milk advocates, coming as it did against the huge empire that was the state of California.

Yet within twenty-four hours of this victory, it seemed as if the state—this time in the form of the federal government—struck back. Armed agents of the FDA paid visits to two of Organic Pastures' low-level employees at their homes after work. I described the situation in a March 20, 2008, blog posting:

> Mark McAfee had just a few hours to celebrate yesterday's issuance of a temporary restraining order blocking enforcement of AB 1735—what he called "a big win for California raw milk and producers"—before he learned about the next phase of the government's campaign against Organic Pastures Dairy Co.

It seems the US Justice Department, in cooperation with the Food and Drug Administration, is conducting a grand jury investigation into OPDC's sales of raw milk and colostrum sold as pet food to consumers around the country, outside of California. Two of OPDC's employees have in the last two weeks each received a subpoena to testify in early April before a US District Court grand jury for the Eastern District of California.

The employees, who take phone orders and help administer the dairy's office, didn't know what the subpoenas were for until after dinner last evening—just hours after the state superior court issued its temporary restraining order on AB 1735—when they received visits at their homes from two FDA special agents from its Office of Criminal Investigations.

In each case, the agents telephoned first, saying they were following up on the subpoenas, and then showed badges before asking to come into the employees' homes and question them. The situation bears an eerie resemblance to the visit by New York agriculture agents to Meadowsweet Dairy within hours of owners Barb and Steve Smith filing suit against the state last December.

Before I relate what the employees say happened next, I should say that I called one of the FDA special agents, Stephen Jackson, on his cell phone, obtained from the business card he left behind. After I identified myself and told him I was inquiring into the grand jury investigation into OPDC, he said, "I'd prefer you not call this number." I then asked him if he could refer me to an FDA or Justice Department official who might be able to help me, but he said he couldn't, and suggested I just call the main number of the US Attorney's office in Fresno.

One of the employees, Amanda Hall, who has worked for OPDC for about a year, said Jackson and his colleague kept inquiring into the sale of raw milk to customers outside California. "They kept saying, 'Do you know it's illegal to sell raw milk outside California?'" When she explained that the milk is labeled as pet food and thus okay, "They said, 'Who told you that?' I said I learned it from others in the office. . . . They kept asking me if I knew it was illegal. . . . At first they were nice and polite, but they kept getting more agitated. I think they wanted to hear about Mark."

There was more to come. One of the agents played a tape recording of Amanda taking a phone order from an FDA agent posing as a customer, inquiring whether it was okay for the "customer's" eight-month-old child to consume colostrum. "I said it was okay. The FDA has no regulations on colostrum. It's a dietary supplement. And all products are labeled for pet consumption."

And then even more: Before the agents left, "One of them asked me, 'Would you ever consider wearing a wire? If you would wear it, you would be getting information from Mark. You could benefit. You wouldn't be paid millions, but it would sure help you out.'" Amanda declined, and the agent left a card, saying that if she changed her mind, she should call.

The situation was pretty similar for Lizbeth Eugenia Valdes-Urbieta, who has been at OPDC for two years, except the visit seems to have been more traumatic for her than for Amanda. "I'm pregnant, and I'm a crybaby," she says. Not only that, her husband, mother, and father were present in the house, and her mother was becoming ever more frightened as she heard the agents pressing their questions. "She asked my husband, 'Is this legal?' He told her it was."

They went through the routine about it being illegal to sell raw milk outside California, she says, "And they told me, 'Don't worry, you're not in trouble.' Then they had a tape of me talking to a customer. He asked me if we ship outside California. He told me he had a son, one year old, and can he drink colostrum?" She says she told him that the children of OPDC employees consume colostrum. "They kept asking me, 'Who told you about the pet food labels?'"

Maybe because she was so nervous, they didn't ask her to wear a wire. "After they left, I was shaking," Lizbeth says.

Mark says he had extensive communication with FDA officials about his pet food labeling back in 2003 and 2004, and that the agency eventually sent him an advisory in early 2005 stating that "there is no requirement that pet food products have premarket approval by the FDA."

One last note: Grand jury investigations are normally secret events in which prosecutors try to convince jurors to vote criminal indictments. Witnesses who are subpoenaed have no right to have a lawyer present and can expect to be cross-examined by a skilled government attorney. The identities of jurors are kept secret as well. Mark says he and his employees decided to go public about the grand jury situation after a meeting this morning of the dairy's dozen employees. "We're a family here," he told me. "We're going to protect ourselves. Our only weapon is the truth."

But he added that he's being practical as well. "I'm ready for a raid right now. All the computers are backed up."

His theory for the government's latest action: "Our sales are going through the roof. We're doing $100,000 a week in sales—last quarter, it was $75,000. People are going nuts for raw milk. The FDA is going nuts the other way. I'm the snake. They want to cut off the head of the snake."

Strange coincidence, these night-time visits by special agents to individuals' homes, just after OPDC wins a big court case. It's a good thing Mark isn't paranoid. He might otherwise think there were people out to get him.[23]

Despite the temporary-restraining-order victory in March, the reality was that Organic Pastures and Claravale, along with their defender, the Farm-to-Consumer Legal Defense Fund, were skating on thin ice. As I've noted before, judges don't like to rule against the state, especially in cases seeming to involve public safety and public welfare. That's why most requests for search warrants are granted. Moreover, getting temporary restraining orders transformed into temporary injunctions requires convincing a judge that your case is strong enough that you could win in a full trial.

Mark McAfee understood this reality, so as part of his campaign to have AB 1735 changed by the California Assembly in January, he had made some additional political contacts. One was with a fast-rising senator, Dean Florez, who was chairman of the state senate's Food Safety Committee. The contact had come about via one of those strange circuitous routes that sometimes present themselves when least expected.

A recent Organic Pastures customer, Christine Chessen, a San Francisco mother of three young children, had begun the previous fall to appreciate the benefits of raw milk once she saw that her children seemed to have fewer colds and other illnesses. She realized when she saw some TV footage of Senator Florez speaking about food-borne illness that the two of them had been college classmates at the University of California–Los Angeles fifteen years earlier.

"On a whim, I decided last fall to write Dean Florez," she told me. "To my surprise, he answered my letter."

His original attitude was concern about "how dangerous" raw milk is, she remembered. "Like a lot of legislators, it was a matter of educating him. . . . They tend to react to stories of kids getting sick and dying from food-borne illness."

She stayed in touch with Senator Florez, and arranged in early 2008 for him to tour Mark McAfee's dairy. He seemed to learn his lessons well, and became not only more accepting of raw milk but also critical of the CDFA's campaign against it.

In mid-April, some weeks before the judge in the court suit was due to rule on the temporary injunction, Florez scheduled a day of hearings about replacing AB 1735. I decided to fly out to California to attend the session. Among other things, I would at long last get to meet Mark McAfee, whom I had known only via phone conversations and e-mails up to this point.

The energy outside the white Capitol in Sacramento that warm and sunny April afternoon was high, given that the number of raw milk supporters was fairly small—perhaps two hundred people. But everyone was enthusiastic, and ordinary consumers were clearly encouraged by the outsiders who had traveled long distances—Sally Fallon Morell of the Weston A. Price Foundation (based in Washington, DC); Michael Schmidt, a Canadian raw milk dairyman whose farm had been raided by authorities there some months earlier because he operated a herd share for Toronto-area consumers; Ted Beals, the Michigan pathologist who provided expert testimony in the raw dairy suit; and Liz Reitzig, a Maryland raw milk activist—not to mention yours truly.

For six hours, consumers and scientists testified about the advantages and disadvantages of raw milk, as Senator Florez proved to be quite the expert. Here is how I described the hearing in my blog posting for April 16, 2008:

> Now that I've had a few hours to reflect, I feel reasonably confident that something will come out of the California hearing. However, it won't be a repeal of the 10-coliform-per-milliliter standard of AB1735. Sen. Dean Florez, who chaired yesterday's California Senate hearing on raw milk, said as much on several occasions.
>
> Perhaps most dramatically, he asked a group of five scientific experts at the conclusion of their testimony in favor of raw milk, "What should be put on the governor's desk?"
>
> One of the experts stated, "Go back to what it was."
>
> Sen. Florez shot back, "It is not going back to the way it was. It is going to be a tougher standard."

Now, at first glance, that sounds ominous. But as the hearing proceeded over a period of six hours, it became clear that Sen. Florez has thought about the process very carefully, and appreciates that, politically, it is impossible to simply repeal AB1735, since that already failed in the California Assembly in January.

What he envisions is a replacement of AB1735 with something that appears tougher to germ-frightened legislators, but is in fact more reasonable for producers. Later in his questioning of the pro-raw-milk experts, he stated, "Why don't we talk about pathogen testing and HACCP [Hazard Analysis and Critical Control Point plan]? At the end of the day, [raw milk] is a different product. I'm just trying to figure out a better test that comes to a standard. But we're not going back to the way it was. We're going to strengthen the standard and then we are going to the pasteurized milk industry and doing the same thing there." That last line elicited strong applause from the 200 or so supporters in the audience.

Sen. Florez in his questioning of experts pro and con, along with the producers—Mark McAfee of Organic Pastures Dairy Co. and Collette Cassidy (co-owner with her husband Ron Garthwaite) of Claravale Farm—continually returned to the themes of HACCP and pathogen testing. (HACCP involves developing a highly structured production process, which can be audited, to reduce the risk of food contamination.) The area where he showed the most uncertainty was over the specifics of a coliform standard—whether it should be increased from 10 to possibly 50 or 100, or whether it can be dispensed with entirely.

He explicitly invited the experts in favor of raw milk to help. "I would encourage you to conference call and produce a bill for Sen. [Edward] Vincent and me that is stronger than a single test. I am asking you to go a step further for us. Determine how Claravale and Organic Pastures can be the leaders in raw milk. . . . Agriculture has a lot of sway in this building. . . . Our raw milk dairies don't have political clout. We're trying to allow raw milk dairies to have political clout."

Mark McAfee suggested he was quite receptive to the senator's suggested approach. "I am very comfortable with HACCP," he said. He pointed out that he already has a "basic" HACCP program in place that he had used when growing apples, though Sen. Florez prodded him to go further. "You say you have a basic HACCP plan. Are you ready to do a world-class HACCP plan?"

Mark said he was prepared to accept a plan that could be audited by outsiders, though "not the state. It all has to do with the mindset of the participants." He also pointed out he is already testing OPDC's milk for key pathogens on a regular basis.

While Mark said he was open to a coliform standard of 50 coliforms per milliliter, Colleen said she wasn't. "Even with 50, we wouldn't pass consistently."

What encourages me that Sen. Florez is serious is that he was talking in terms of specific items that could be included within legislation, and what compromises might be possible. Politicians are usually more serious at that stage than when they wax eloquent about broad generalities.

It was also clear he appreciates the urgency created by the lawsuit filed by OPDC and Claravale against the California Department of Food and Agriculture (in which a judge granted a temporary restraining order against enforcing AB1735). He asked Colleen about the suit, and she answered that it was only filed when Claravale and OPDC were pushed close to the brink of shutting down. "It's preferable to have a legislative solution [rather] than a court solution," she told Sen. Florez.

Sen. Florez was clearly very pissed at CDFA for not being there, and even asked Mark and Colleen what they thought. Mark wisely took the high road, saying "I'm very disappointed. They have a lot to add."

After the hearing, I asked Sen. Florez what else might happen because of CDFA's refusal to send a representative. "We're not done with that," he told me. "We're going to ask the governor's office to look into it."

And has the senator become a raw milk convert? No, he said, he doesn't drink it. "I'm trying to remain neutral," he said. He added that hearing from his old classmate, Christine Chessen, last fall, "inspired me to try to get a better standard." Left unsaid is that he's being talked about as a future candidate for lieutenant governor.[24]

For raw milk proponents favoring a change to AB 1735, Senator Florez's involvement turned out to be quite fortuitous, because at a court hearing in May, the judge refused to issue a preliminary injunction in the dairies' suit, and told the plaintiffs that the preferable way to settle the entire matter would be through the original source of the problem: the California legislature. Since things were already moving along well in that arena, the focus shifted there, and would stay there for the next six months.

Within days of the hearing, members of Senator Florez's staff were on the phone with Mark McAfee, who had returned to his dairy in Fresno, seeking his input in drafting new legislation that would essentially substitute a HACCP-based plan for the coliform standard.

According to a digest on the legislature's Web site, SB 201:

> This bill would provide alternative requirements for dairy farms that produce and process guaranteed raw milk, or Grade A raw milk, to be sold to the consumer and would state that dairy farms choosing to comply with the alternative requirements do not have to comply with those existing requirements. Specifically, under the alternative requirements, this bill would require a dairy farm that produces and processes raw milk, as defined, to develop and maintain an individualized Hazard Analysis Critical Control Point plan for each critical process in the production of raw milk on the dairy farm, and would require the plan to be approved by the Department of Food and Agriculture and the State Department of Public Health, as specified.[25]

By substituting the HACCP process for the coliform standard, SB 201 seemed to take the air out of the food safety histrionics that had surrounded AB 1735. In late August, SB 201 gained approval of the California Assembly by a unanimous vote, and then a week later by a 33–4 vote in the Senate. Next stop: the governor's desk.

It wouldn't have been California if there weren't some additional fireworks, however. When actor Martin Sheen appeared together with Senator Florez and Mark McAfee at a press conference in early September outside a Whole Foods store in Venice to support SB 201, and drank from a jug of Organic Pastures milk, opponents from a food blog carrying signs, VETO SB 201, shouted at Sheen and Florez. It made great copy for their blog.[26]

All this was on top of the YouTube video showing Chris Martin, the seven-year-old boy who was thought to have been sickened by Organic Pastures raw milk, on life support (which I described in chapter 9). That video was removed after Mark McAfee's lawyer protested to the Martin family's lawyer, Bill Marler, a prominent personal injury lawyer who specializes in food-borne illness cases.

However, Marler wasn't about to walk away with his tail between his legs. In late August, he published a blog posting, headed, "Gov. Schwarzenegger, Veto This Bill!" In it he relied heavily on the fear-laden images of sick children:

> It's difficult to work so hard against a bill that has such good intentions. But SB 201 actually creates a detour around the regulation of raw milk, and must be re-written before the bill is ready. There are children on life support because of raw milk tainted with E. *coli* and other toxic bacteria, and there will be more of them in California—and nationwide—unless changes are made to this legislation.[27]

I was inclined to dismiss the article out of hand—what the heck, Marler is just another personal injury attorney out there. But the reality is that he isn't just another personal injury lawyer. He's a very marketing-savvy lawyer who had done a brilliant job using blogs to further his practice and, in the process, established himself as the biggest name in food-borne illness cases. In that role, he had gained considerable influence in state departments of public health and agriculture, where officials often sympathized with his tough line on food safety.

These officials sometimes even benefit financially from his damage suits on behalf of individuals who have become seriously ill from food-borne illness, when they are retained by him as expert witnesses. For example, in the cases of Chris Martin and Lauren Herzog, he assembled expert witness statements from six public health experts, all of whom are, or have been, senior public health officials in Oregon, Minnesota, and Washington State, and at the US Centers for Disease Control. I'm not suggesting there is anything improper in any of this—just explaining how it is Marler could write the letter he wrote and expect that agriculture and public health advisers to the governor might bring it to his attention.[28]

So the big question became this: Would Governor Schwarzenegger be listening?

CHAPTER TWELVE

A Test of Belief Systems

As various battles brewed over raw milk—in Michigan, Ohio, New York, Pennsylvania, and California—I very nearly forgot about the incident (described in chapter 1) that had originally piqued my curiosity about raw milk. That was the case of Dee Creek Farm in Washington State, which flared up in late 2005 after a number of adults and children—part of a raw milk herd share set up by the farm owners—were sickened by *E. coli* O157:H7.

Every once in a while, Pete Kennedy of the Farm-to-Consumer Legal Defense Fund would call me with updates about the latest legal issue confronting Dee Creek. It seemed as if Kennedy was continually trying to placate and negotiate with aggressive prosecutors—but he always ended with the admonition: "I don't think you should write about it quite yet. It's still dicey." In other words, my writing about the case in the midst of legal posturing could complicate matters for the owners; as much as I wanted to update my blog readers about this mysterious raw milk situation, I always placed the legal welfare of the owners of the small dairies first in the sense of trying to avoid making their sometimes precarious situations worse by irritating regulators and prosecutors.

And dicey the Dee Creek situation was, as became crystal clear in September 2008. That was when the case was finally resolved in a federal court via a plea agreement, with the judge taking the highly unusual step of reducing the agreed-upon penalty and reprimanding prosecutors for having gone overboard in their pursuit of the owners.

Here is what I wrote about the case and its resolution, under the heading, "How Much Punishment Is Enough for a Couple's Tainted Raw Milk? A Federal Judge Finally Decides":

> If you want to know how serious the US government is about dis-
> couraging raw milk consumption, especially via herd shares, con-
> sider the experiences of Anita and Michael Puckett, owners of Dee
> Creek Farm in Washington state.

Dee Creek is the dairy whose raw milk apparently sickened anywhere between seven and eighteen of its shareholders—depending on whose version you believe—with *E. coli* O157:H7 back in December 2005. The two most seriously ill were children who developed HUS (hemolytic uremic syndrome) and had to be hospitalized for a month. They recovered, as did everyone else.

I've been trying to report on the situation with Dee Creek since early 2006, but because of the Pucketts' legal problems, have held off. Even after I learned last November about the fact that the US Justice Department was seeking a criminal indictment against the Pucketts, I was requested by a lawyer representing the Pucketts to delay any reporting, since it could worsen their situation. Earlier this week, though, the legal case finally came to a conclusion, and Anita's sister, Katrina Florence, released a number of legal documents relating to the case.

These documents show that between the illnesses and the notification from the Justice Department about the possible criminal indictment, Anita and her husband, Michael, together with the help of friends and insurance coverage, paid state penalties to the Washington State Department of Agriculture of $8,000, plus $70,000 to children who became ill from Dee Creek milk. That doesn't count the $15,000 it cost them to keep feeding their cows over more than a year, nor many months of lost income from not being able to distribute their milk.

The US Justice Department's notice (that its "investigation has developed substantial evidence linking you to the commission of a crime, and that, in the judgment of this office, you are a putative defendant in a criminal case") arrived just at a time when the Pucketts thought they were finally putting this nightmare behind them.

Keep in mind, the Pucketts made their milk available under a herd-share agreement, so the federal government was coming after them because some of their share owners lived over the border in Oregon. It wasn't even as if the Pucketts delivered the milk over the border, and it wasn't as if the Pucketts were selling milk. As part of the herd-share agreements they signed, the shareowners all agreed that they understood the potential dangers of raw milk.

After some months of negotiation between the US attorney's

office and the Pucketts, the US attorney's office, in all its magnanimity, agreed to recommend to a judge that the Pucketts be given a year of probation if they would plead guilty to their crimes. This wasn't a guarantee, though. According to the plea agreement, the Pucketts "knowingly introduced, or aided and abetted the introduction, of food into interstate commerce" and "Second, the food was prepared, packed or held under unsanitary conditions whereby it may have been rendered injurious to health." The judge could have sentenced the Pucketts to up to a year in prison, a fine of up to $100,000, and up to one year of supervision after release from jail.

The Pucketts, who were out of money and in debt, as well as emotionally exhausted, agreed to the deal.

In a letter to the court, here is how they described their experiences after shareholders became ill:

> The first couple of months were spent with a dark, oppressive "cloud" hanging over us for fear for the children. Anita could only sleep for moments at a time, waking to crushing feelings of horror and panic. She could not eat. She could not think. She could not speak. She could not even pray, except for mercy for those kids.
>
> Anita began experiencing a full-time "anxiety attack." At first she was in a state of shock, then constantly crying. She became inconsolable, debilitated; unable to cope with everyday life. We did not pay our bills, or take care of necessary business. Anita refused to take or make telephone calls except with ill co-owners, becoming terrified of what every ringing telephone might bring. She paced from room to room. Whenever a moment opened up where thoughts came flooding in, she would involuntarily moan and wail. Her blood pressure shot up, and she began experiencing heart palpitations and hyperventilation. Her physician put her on blood pressure medication and referred her for counseling.
>
> For several months, we became wary of the safety of any food. Anita went through a period of paranoia, worrying about everything that went into our children's

mouths. We obsessively checked everyone's stools for many months following.

When we managed to survive the WSDA issues, then the civil settlement, we began to think life might return to its pre-chaotic state. The shock of a criminal prosecution was almost too much to bear. We are very patriotic people, and it hurt to see "United States of America" vs. ourselves. The "criminal" label has been a very heavy burden, especially to Anita and her self-image, so much so that she has returned to counseling. Her therapist has suggested that Prozac might be in order for her.

Our children have suffered. [The Pucketts have four grown children and seven adopted children living at home.] As result of media harassment, our children have become nervous of helicopters, airplanes, police, reporters, and the legal system.

There has been great personal financial devastation. We have barely survived these almost three years. Earlier this year our house/farm went into foreclosure. Thankfully, friends lent us the money to get it out. . . . Our credit has been destroyed.

Last Friday, the Pucketts appeared before federal magistrate judge Karen L. Strombom in Tacoma, who heard the recommendation . . . and refused to go along with the deal. Here's what she said:

"I frankly don't see what benefit anybody gets from putting these people on probation. I realize everybody here has come to this court agreeing to that, but I don't agree with it."

She accepted the guilty plea to a Class A misdemeanor as "sufficient punishment," adding: "I don't see how we accomplish anything by having these two people put on probation. I just don't get it."

Just for emphasis, she gave the Pucketts six months to pay off a $25 special assessment she was required to impose.

As admirable as Judge Strombom's words and decision might be, it is, unfortunately, too little, too late. The message has gone out loud and clear from the US government. The Pucketts have certainly gotten the message. They are currently milking 35 goats and making cheese that they age for 60 days, under US Food and Drug Administration requirements. They sell the cheese at farmers markets. No more raw milk sales, and no more herd-share arrangements for them, and you can understand why.

But the couple included this warning in their statement to the court:

"There appears to be an upward spiral of contaminated food incidents occurring in the full spectrum of available food, with grave illnesses contracted, even deaths. Pathogenic outbreaks occur daily. Singling out a very small producer to be one of the first in criminal prosecution involving food-borne illness, fosters discouragement to small farmers everywhere."

Unfortunately, that is exactly the intent.[1]

The federal magistrate had raised a most interesting question, though: Why was this case being pursued so aggressively? In fact, the same question could be asked about a number of the cases I have covered in this book. The questioning by armed FDA agents of Organic Pastures' two employees one day after a state judge had issued a temporary restraining order in the AB 1735 challenge (described in the previous chapter) had finally led to a criminal indictment of both the company and its owner, Mark McAfee, in late 2008. The main charge: selling raw milk across state lines, in violation of a federal prohibition. Within months, McAfee had agreed to a plea deal whereby he would refrain from selling raw milk via mail to out-of-staters, rather than spend many thousands of dollars trying to defend himself in court.[2] (An FDA civil suit against Organic Pastures in connection with the interstate sales of colostrums, and objections to claims for raw milk made on the dairy's Web site, remained outstanding, however.[3])

And then there were the big-state cases still outstanding—the one pitting Meadowsweet Dairy against the New York Department of Agriculture and Markets (described in chapter 10) and the challenge to AB 1735 by Organic Pastures and Claravale in California. (Even though a judge refused to issue a preliminary injunction in May 2008, and encouraged a legislative resolution, the suit was still active and pending.)

The federal cases, and quite possibly a number of the state cases as well, were apparently being pushed by the US Food and Drug Administration, in particular by the head of its Division of Plant and Dairy Food Safety, John

Sheehan. He's the man I had taken to referring to on my blog as "the Milk Czar."

He is also the man best known for the statement, "Drinking raw milk or eating raw milk products is like playing Russian roulette with your health."[4]

Thus, in both actions and words, Sheehan was adamantly opposed to any flexibility or permissiveness at all concerning raw milk. It's worse than that, though. Sheehan has made clear on any number of occasions that he is also completely opposed to any kind of dialogue with raw milk advocates, to the extent he can't stand to be in the same room, or even the same building, as them. On top of that, he turned out to be an elusive, almost a mysterious, bureaucrat.

I tried on any number of occasions to arrange some kind of a meeting or interview with the man . . . and eventually began to feel almost obsessive about it. When finally I did meet him, I described it in a blog posting this way:

> I'm almost embarrassed to admit that I traveled 2,500 miles in large measure to snap a photo of a reclusive bureaucrat.
>
> Here's the story. For many months I've been trying to obtain information about John Sheehan, director of the US Food and Drug Administration's Division of Plant and Dairy Food Safety. I've taken to referring to him as the nation's Milk Czar, since he has been orchestrating much of the anti-raw-milk activity that's been going on around the country the last few years, and is notable for his frequent quote, "Drinking raw milk is like playing Russian roulette with your health."
>
> Early this year (2009), I made a formal request of FDA to interview him in connection with the book I am writing about raw milk. No surprise—I was turned down. But what was curious to me was that the agency provided only the sketchiest of biographical information.
>
> In its six sentences, it said Sheehan was a patent lawyer who joined the FDA in 2000 after serving as "a mid-level manager within the dairy industry for 17 years. He has worked for some of America's largest and most progressive dairy foods organizations." When I asked for the names of these "most progressive dairy foods organizations," the FDA refused to provide them. It also said it had no photograph of him.

If you do a Google search on Sheehan, you don't find much. Nothing about his career, and no photos. (There was one site that supposedly had photos of him at a dairy gathering in Poland, but there were two different guys identified as Sheehan.)

Then, in February, I went to the raw milk symposium outside Washington sponsored by the International Association for Food Protection, where Sheehan was scheduled to be a speaker, expecting to meet him. Lo and behold, I was told he canceled out the Friday before without giving a reason. (An FDA spokesperson later said he didn't attend because there is outstanding litigation—wouldn't say what—but presumably a civil suit still pending against Organic Pastures Dairy Co.)

By this time, I'm beginning to wonder: Is this guy for real, or just a fun-loving figment of the bureaucracy's imagination? So when I heard about the gathering of the National Conference on Interstate Milk Shipments being held this weekend in Orlando, I figured what the heck, let's give it another shot. Yes, I did also want to see Mark McAfee of Organic Pastures make his pitch for lifting the ban on interstate shipments of raw milk.

But this thing with Sheehan was becoming something of an obsession. Sheehan didn't attend Mark McAfee's presentation early this morning, but an associate of his, Cindy Leonard, the presenter of the notorious 2005 FDA slide presentation that slams raw milk, was on the committee hearing the McAfee proposal.

Afterwards, I tried to engage Leonard, but she refused, saying there was litigation that prevented her from commenting, and she walked away from me. A few minutes later, I saw her in the hallway, and tried again, saying I just wanted to ask her about the Division of Dairy and Plant Food Safety. This time, she turned and actually started running from me, which was a tad awkward, since she was wearing high heels.

But at a general session following McAfee's presentation, I got someone to point out my real prey, John Sheehan. I had to listen to a lengthy presentation about parliamentary rules, but finally, I got my chance. I decided to snap my photos first, before engaging him in conversation. I wish I could say Sheehan was being cute by putting a notebook in front of his face, but I don't think he was. A photo [he allowed to be taken immediately thereafter] I think was just an effort on his part to keep from embarrassing himself in front of the other people there. The reason I don't think he's being funny is because this was my conversation with Sheehan after taking the photos:

"Hi, I'm David Gumpert."

"Yes, I know who you are."

"I wonder if we could chat for just a few moments."

"No."

"Why not?"

"Because I don't want to."

Well, you have to give the guy credit for being honest. No more funny stuff about "pending litigation." He just doesn't want to be f***ing bothered. If a guy doesn't want to talk to you, there's not much you can do, even if you do help pay his salary. But at least I do know one thing: John Sheehan really does exist.[5]

The FDA's tough and secretive approach in its anti-raw-milk campaign is ironic because, not that long ago, it was accused by consumer advocates of being too easy on raw milk, of shying away from banning raw milk in interstate commerce. During the early 1980s, when the availability of raw milk was entirely a matter of state regulation, a consumer group formed by Ralph Nader and Public Citizen (interesting because Nader is California's Green Party leader—big on organics, global warming, et cetera) became convinced that the FDA should clamp down. When the FDA failed to respond the way Public Citizen wanted—with a ban on interstate sales of raw milk—the organization filed suit in federal court. An official of Public Citizen was quoted in *The New York Times* as claiming that "since 1980 there have been more than 1,000 cases of human infection and more than 20 deaths from drinking unpasteurized milk, certified or not." ("Certified" raw milk had the approval of the American Association of Medical Milk Commissions, which was a quasi-regulatory organization established in the early 1900s to oversee the production of safe raw milk around the country.)[6]

The frustration felt by those medical and public health officials who thought the federal government should have clamped down in advance of a suit being filed is expressed as well by the rabidly anti-raw-milk Web site Quackwatch. "The FDA had stayed a proposed ban in 1973 and had begun to draft regulations again in 1982, but stalled until prodded by Public Citizen's health research group (HRG). HRG petitioned the agency in April

1984 and, together with the American Public Health Association (APHA), filed suit in September 1984 to force a response."[7]

Another anti-raw-milk group, which I quoted in the previous chapter in relation to the Alta Dena dairy producing raw milk in California, summarized the dynamics more colorfully:

> In 1984, Public Citizen Health Research Group petitioned the FDA to ban interstate distribution of CRM as a public health danger, but Alta Dena also had friends in Washington. Congressman William Dannemeyer was Alta Dena's General Counsel, and Ronald Reagan was a California Republican with a strong anti-regulatory agenda—even in matters affecting public health. Reagan's HHS Secretary, Margaret Heckler, prevented FDA from acting. Public Citizen then sued Heckler and won. This resulted in a 1987 federal court order directing the FDA to institute a ban (the judge found that Heckler had acted in an "arbitrary and capricious" manner by disregarding public health data on the risks of raw milk.[8]

It's interesting as well to read on that same Quackwatch Web page an account of hearings held before the FDA in 1984, after Public Citizen had filed its suit. According to the article, by a freelance writer, proponent after proponent testified on behalf of raw milk. There were citizens questioning the public health intentions of authorities, a pediatrician saying that his patients' health was better with raw milk, and a physician who maintained that pasteurized milk was "dead milk, which will rot on standing."

It's difficult to imagine John Sheehan chairing such a hearing today, even if the outcome was preordained against raw milk. He obviously can't even stand to be in close proximity to people who favor consumption of raw milk, so adamantly opposed is he.

When I began work on this book, I happened to meet up with a classmate and good friend of mine from my days as an undergraduate at the University of Chicago, Michael Seidman. I asked Mike, a professor for many years specializing in constitutional law at Georgetown University Law School,[9] about Article 1, Section 10 of the US Constitution, the so-called Contract Clause, which states, "No State shall . . . pass . . . **a Law impairing the Obligation of Contracts**, or grant any Title of Nobility" (boldface emphasis added).[10] Wouldn't this explicit statement protect herd-share arrangements, whereby consumers enter into a private contractual arrangement with dairy farmers to financially support the dairy herd in exchange for a regular supply of milk?

Mike laughed, as if his old college buddy was really out of it. The Contract Clause had pretty much been eviscerated over the years, he explained, by government arguments about the public welfare, or protection of public health, needing to take precedence.

I would receive direct confirmation of his assessment during the summer and fall of 2008, when two decisions were issued in connection with Meadowsweet Dairy. This was the New York dairy that established a limited liability company (LLC) as a type of herd share; I described its legal fight against the New York Department of Agriculture and Markets in chapter 10. Under the LLC arrangement, consumers essentially entered into private contracts to obtain raw dairy products from Meadowsweet, outside the public regulatory structure of NY Ag & Markets.

But two legal arbiters would have none of it. First, in August 2008, the hearing officer engaged by the agency, who oversaw the two days of hearings in January 2008, issued her ruling, which I described on my blog:

> The notion that a hearing officer engaged by New York's Department of Agriculture and Markets would recommend a ruling in favor of the agency, and against Barb and Steve Smith, is no big surprise. What is surprising is the logic the officer, Susan Weber, used in her 21-page report—just sent last week to the Smiths—which is based on two days of hearings held last January concerning charges against the Smiths and their Meadowsweet Dairy LLC. The Smiths established a limited liability company—really, a type of herd share— and argued that the LLC placed them outside the tentacles of NY Ag & Markets.
>
> Even less of a surprise is that the Ag & Markets Commissioner, Patrick Hooker, accepted the hearing officer's recommendations and ordered the Smiths to abide by state regulations, including obtaining a raw milk permit, if they want to make unpasteurized milk available to their shareholders. Of course, that would mean they couldn't make other products like yogurt, cream, butter, and buttermilk available. Hooker actually went further than the hearing officer, ignoring even her two modestly favorable findings for the Smiths: that no raw-milk sales had occurred, and that the Smiths' milk hadn't violated coliform standards, since none exist in New York for raw milk.

What's interesting about Weber's report is that it seems to be telling the Smiths: You may be doing everything correctly in using an LLC to distribute milk to shareholders, but it's illegal all the same.

For example, to the argument by the Smiths' lawyer, Gary Cox (of the Farm-to-Consumer Legal Defense Fund) that New York's milk laws don't prohibit herd-share–type arrangements, hearing officer Weber states: "There is the definition of raw milk, which appears to require a sale; there is the consumer who must apparently purchase in order for the milk she or he drinks to be regulated under law; there is the milk plant which must apparently receive milk intended for pasteurization or not qualify as a milk plant. Respondents would have us hang our hats upon these inconsistencies, find them dispositive, and dismiss the State's case. To do so would fly in the face of common sense and defeat the clear legislative intent to cover the field of dairy regulation for the protection of public health."

Yes, "protection" over all.

Similarly, she states: "I conclude that the arrangement between its members and Meadowsweet for the distribution of raw milk and raw milk products is not a purchase and sale transaction, but is a distribution of profit based upon the value of the members' contributions."

But then she adds, "It is well established that the law cannot be employed for an illegal purpose. . . . Consequently, while members may obtain raw milk and raw milk products at the farm as a distribution from the LLC, I find that the LLC must be in compliance with applicable laws governing manufacture, processing, handling, and distribution of dairy products."

Shades of *Catch-22*?

Finally, she expresses concerns about sanitation violations discovered by Ag & Markets, including "the north wall is caked with old manure, chickens were found roaming free in the milking barn," along with flies, mouse droppings, and spider webs observed. Even though she allows that "the Department offered no evidence that there was any actual injury to the public or any intent to deceive consumers by offering product which was not what it was purported to be," the claim about unsanitary conditions "was the most compelling" to her.

To Weber, "The Department's evidence establishes beyond doubt that the conditions at Meadowsweet in October of 2007 were not sanitary, that the products produced, processed and manufactured there may have been contaminated with filth or rendered diseased, unwholesome or injurious to health."

Never mind that real farms have for ages had chickens intermingling with cows, and have had spider webs and mouse droppings around . . . or that no members of the LLC-herd share have become ill, or even made a single complaint to any governmental authorities, after numerous visits to the dairy to pick up their milk.

It's easy to dismiss this report as inherently biased and also point out that it isn't yet enforceable because the Smiths have a court case pending against Ag & Markets in state court seeking exemption from Ag & Markets of the LLC–herd-share model.

But the fact is that a quasi-legal opinion has moved the nation's second-largest state a large step closer to rendering herdshares illegal. You can be sure the judge in the Smiths' case will read the hearing officer's report. This New York decision comes after a court in the nation's largest state sided with the California Department of Food and Agriculture a few months ago in refusing to suspend enforcement of the state's 10-coliform-per-milliliter coliform standard.

In both cases, the voices of the judiciary were essentially saying: You raw-milk people may have logical arguments, but we mortal judge types don't pretend to really understand this stuff, so we're accepting everything the regulators tell us, whether it's true or not, because . . . they're regulators and, doggone it, we trust them to protect our health. And you few who don't trust them to protect your health, well, that's your problem.[11]

Then a state judge, who had heard the court case filed by the Farm-to-Consumer Legal Defense Fund on behalf of Meadowsweet, issued a not dissimilar decision from the Ag & Markets hearing officer in November 2008.

In a blunt decision issued Thursday that no doubt has the tough guys at the New York Department of Agriculture and Markets doing high-fives, state judge John C. Egan Jr. sided completely with the agency in its long-running feud with Meadowsweet Dairy LLC, and owners Barb and Steve Smith. The Smiths set up a limited liability company to serve the herd-share role for 120-plus shareholders in the Ithaca, New York, area, who wanted access to such unpasteurized dairy products as yogurt, butter, and cream, which are prohibited for dairies that obtain raw milk permits from the state. NY Ag & Markets didn't take well to the idea of a small dairy operating outside its grasp, nor of setting a precedent that other dairies might look to.

The immediate issue was Meadowsweet's request for a preliminary injunction to prohibit NY Ag & Markets from conducting seemingly arbitrary searches of the dairy and seizures of Meadowsweet's products, and to allow the LLC's members regular access to their products. At one point, NY Ag & Markets threatened to lock the couple up.

The judge essentially ruled against each argument offered by Meadowsweet's lawyer, Gary Cox of the Farm-to-Consumer Legal Defense Fund.

- To the Meadowsweet argument that the state's arbitrary seizures of raw dairy products threatened to put the dairy out of business, the judge stated: ". . . the Court finds the plaintiffs' allegations that they 'run the risk of' losing product, being searched at any time and having their personal belongings seized at any time, speculative. Furthermore, any financial injuries sustained as a result of the loss of product do not establish irreparable harm. Thus, the plaintiffs have failed to establish irreparable harm . . ." Guess he thinks they have a money tree in the backyard to keep replacing the thousands of dollars worth of product NY Ag & Markets doused with bleach.

- To the Meadowsweet argument that its limited liability company should be outside the regulation and arbitrary inspections of NY Ag and Markets, the judge stated: "The Commissioner is entitled to full access to Meadowsweet, and may also examine and open any package or container of any kind . . ." In other words, NY Ag and Markets can conduct searches whenever it wants, any time of day or night. Never mind the US Constitution's Fourth Amendment.

- To Meadowsweet's argument that its shareholders aren't purchasing dairy products, and thus aren't "consumers," the judge cited various dictionary definitions of the term "consumer" and concluded: "The Court further determines that the LLC members are 'consumers' of raw milk products based on the plain meaning of the word." So much for Article 1, Section 10 of the US Constitution that "no state shall . . . pass any . . . law impairing the obligation of contracts . . ." (This is the same clause that prohibits use of anything except gold and silver coin as money.)

In sum, the judge fell back on the tired old argument of protection: "Finally, the Court holds that a balancing of the equities weighs in the State's favor, based on the broad powers of the Department of Agriculture and Markets and the State's interest in regulating the dairy industry for the safety of consumers."

Barb and Steve Smith in an email to their shareholders today said, "It seems very possible that we will have to stop distributing raw milk and yogurt . . . and that our friendly inspectors will be watching soon." The Farm-to-Consumer Legal Defense Fund is considering whether to appeal. Given the judge's forceful decision, an appeal would seem to be more of a long shot than ever.

NY Ag & Markets is already licking its chops—in a press release posted Friday the agency indicated its inspectors are already organizing squads "dedicated to administering and enforcing the State's food safety laws and regulations to protect the public health . . ." Yes, I'd say the Smiths can expect visitors.

Clearly, the whole herd-share approach has been called into question. While the concept has received backing in Ohio cases, a negative decision in a major population center and dairy state like New York is a big blow against raw milk.[12]

As it turned out, the Smiths did appeal their case; as of publication of this book, the case remains pending and regulators have not visited them.

If the US Constitution's Contract Clause has now lost its import, what about state legislative authority? In California, following near-unanimous approval of SB 201 (eliminating the coliform standard imposed by AB 1735, described in the previous chapter) by the California Senate and Assembly, raw milk consumers during the fall of 2008 anxiously awaited a decision by Governor Arnold Schwarzenegger.

On September 30, he announced his decision: a veto. Not just a routine veto, but one so harsh in its words, it signaled to his party's legislators that they shouldn't attempt an override:

> Looking past the lobbying techniques, public relations campaign, and legal maneuvering in the courts, one conclusion is inescapably clear: the standard in place has kept harmful products off the shelves and California's raw milk dairies have been operating successfully under it for the entirety of 2008.
>
> Based on fears with no basis in fact, the proponents of SB 201 seek to replace California's unambiguous food safety standards for raw milk. Instead they have created a convoluted and undefined regulatory process with no enforcement authority or clear standards to protect public health. For these reasons, I cannot support this measure.
>
> Sincerely,
>
> Arnold[13]

What raw milk proponents didn't know at the time was that opponents of SB 201 had mounted an intensive campaign aimed at convincing the governor to veto the legislation. The Web site posting by food poisoning lawyer Bill Marler described in the previous chapter ("Gov. Schwarzenegger, Veto This Bill") had apparently been just the tip of the iceberg—more meaningful than SB 201 proponents realized. It apparently signaled that a handful of opponents, with access to the governor, had mobilized themselves to oppose the legislation. It seems very likely, given the timing, that the governor was shown the video of young Chris Martin on life support (mentioned in chapter 9). And dairy industry groups, which had at first supported SB 201, had by this time removed their names from among the list of supporters. In addition, Senator Florez, the chief proponent of the legislation, was a Democrat (Governor Schwarzenegger is a Republican) who was preparing himself for a run at lieutenant governor. Moreover, the governor was in a general pissy mood about a massive state budget crisis, and threatened on more than one occasion to veto lots of legislation (even though SB 201 didn't require any financial support).

Two other California legal matters, the cases of Chris Martin and Lauren Herzog, children allegedly sickened by Organic Pastures milk in September 2006, were settled out of court for undisclosed terms in early 2009.

In light of the pitched legal and legislative battles being fought over raw milk, it's only natural to ask: What is behind the regulators' fervent opposition to raw milk?

I tried to answer this question as I was writing this book. As I noted earlier in this chapter, I began by inviting dairy chief John Sheehan of the FDA to allow me to interview him. When he refused, I went to several of the chief dairy regulators in states that had had the most difficult struggles over raw milk—Michigan, Pennsylvania, California, and New York.

In Michigan, I wanted to explore with Katherine Fedder (mentioned in chapter 1) her reasoning for going after dairy farmer Richard Hebron so aggressively in October 2006. I also wanted to inquire into the progress she had made with a fence-mending committee established after the case settled, known as the Michigan Fresh Unprocessed Whole Milk Workgroup.[14]

But after at first indicating she might be open to speaking with me, in the end she refused, saying blandly, "I do not want to take a chance on compromising any of the work that we are doing here in Michigan."

It was a similar situation in Pennsylvania, where Bill Chirdon, the Pennsylvania Department of Agriculture's director of food safety, had aggressively pursued court cases against Mark Nolt and Glen Wise, seizing thousands of dollars in products and equipment from Nolt in three raids on his farm. I briefly interviewed Chirdon early in 2007 while investigating the Michigan case involving Richard Hebron. The prosecutor in the Michigan case told me he had requested information on a Pennsylvania farmer who was supplying some raw milk cheese products aged less than sixty days (as required by the FDA) to Hebron for sale to members of the Ann Arbor co-op. Such sales are illegal within Pennsylvania, and violate federal law when the cheese is shipped out of state.

Chirdon answered his own phone and seemed very friendly. "I grew up on a large farm in Ohio," he told me by way of background. He had also worked for Dean Foods, a large dairy processor, as a plant manager.

His concerns about raw milk? "With fresh milk, you have to be careful," he said. "Some of these people feel all bacteria are safe. They believe in it. Heating your bacteria doesn't make your milk poisonous."

That conversation in January 2007 was the last one I had with Chirdon, as he, too, refused to be interviewed for this book.

Interestingly, agriculture officials in New York and California didn't turn me down, but they set tough ground rules: I couldn't interview anyone directly, and instead had to submit my questions in writing. Not the most spontaneous approach to interviewing. So here is how one question, relating to possible problems in pathogen testing, which I described in chapter 5, was dealt with by Will Francis, New York's director of milk control and dairy services:

> Q: A number of farms producing raw milk in New York have expressed concern about your findings of listeria in their milk over the last two years. They argue that your policy of shutting down dairies with a finding of as much as a single *Listeria monocytogenes* cell is counter to research suggesting that listeria at very low levels isn't dangerous. They also point out no one has become ill. Are you considering adjusting your testing standards or approach?
>
> A: No.

Or this one:

> Q: What is your position about allowing dairies licensed to sell raw milk to also be able to sell other raw dairy products like yogurt, butter, cream, and other such products?
>
> A. Our current regulations do not allow the sale of raw dairy products, other than raw milk cheese that is aged for at least 60 days.

In California, the approach was much the same, only here I couldn't even attribute the quotes to a particular individual. I had to attribute them to the personable California Department of Food and Agriculture. But no matter. The answers were pretty much as sterile as the ones from New York:

> Q: What are the biggest challenges associated with maintaining the safety of the California raw milk supply, ongoing?
>
> A: As with any food, it's important to produce, handle and package raw milk in a clean and sanitary manner. This is particularly important when the protective step of pasteurization is not employed to eliminate potential foodborne pathogens.

I thought that, since the CDFA is charged with helping farmers succeed financially, I'd try a question related to the business opportunities associated with selling raw milk. But no dice:

> Q: Could encouraging expanded raw milk sales in California be a way to turn around the declining fortunes of conventional dairy farming in California, based on declining prices and rising production of conventional milk?
>
> A: Raw milk is a legal dairy product in California, and may be produced and distributed in accordance with the Food and Agricultural Code. Market demand determines sales declines or increases.

It was clear I'd have to try other tactics if I was going to gain insight into the regulator mentality. One I attempted was convincing a couple of regulators to speak on condition of anonymity. I persuaded a California regulator to be interviewed on these terms, and posted the interview on my blog as a two-part series. This individual's justification for tight controls for raw milk rests largely on the conviction within public health circles that possible health benefits of raw milk are unproven.[15]

During our discussion, it was apparent we had entirely different perspectives on the raw milk conundrum. At one point the individual said, "The scientific evidence on the health benefits are not accepted by the scientific community. Why can't you just pasteurize raw milk?" The individual was truly puzzled.

What about the studies indicating that children who consume raw milk have fewer chronic health problems, such as the recent major European study suggesting that raw milk reduces the incidence of asthma in children? The response: "Isn't it better to go to your doctor and get asthma medicine than to take the risk of drinking raw milk?"

That was a question I wouldn't have even thought to ask. I just assume it's preferable to consume a food to solve a potential health problem than take a powerful pharmaceutical drug or, worse yet, put my child on the drug.

In this individual's view, the basic problem is this: "Raw milk is not stable. You have these illnesses that will happen without controls."

The regulator did allow, though, that the scientific community doesn't fully understand what makes people get ill from pathogens. "It is not just the germs. It is the immune system and you have this interplay. . . . Fifty people go to a banquet and ten get sick."

The regulator also said that public health people are beginning to suspect that raw milk isn't a serious problem for everyone who consumes it. "One of our suspicions is it's the recent drinkers of raw milk who are likeliest to get sick. You develop immunity. It's a natural vaccine. You are self-vaccinating."

This individual feels that the key to improving raw milk's safety is to keep its distribution as local as possible. In this scheme, large operations, like that of Organic Pastures Dairy Co., with hundreds of cows, are the riskiest, since raw milk is a fragile food. "I'd rather it be distributed and regulated locally."

A second regulator, with Wisconsin's Department of Agriculture, Trade and Consumer Protection, was less flexible than the California regulator. "Raw milk is a public health threat," she told me. "We have to keep it under control."

Indeed, this regulator was irritated that her superiors weren't being aggressive enough in a state where raw milk is distributed primarily via herd-share arrangements. She felt as if the herd shares were being allowed to spring up without state oversight. "We haven't had the political will to go after them," she complained.

While the regulators' education and training efforts have conditioned everyone in public health to view raw milk as a huge threat, another factor that tends not to be acknowledged is the role played by the dairy industry. Perhaps because regulators are sensitive to charges of being manipulated by the industry, the ones I spoke with tended to portray the regulatory and dairy industry communities as very much independent of each other.

I've tended to be skeptical, as well, about the charge, made by a number of readers of my blog, that the crackdown on small dairies producing raw milk is somehow an outgrowth of a conspiratorial alliance of between regulators and Big Dairy. Not that I doubt the regulators and dairy industry cooperate in many matters—it's just that I'm not a big believer in conspiracies. In this case, raw milk just seems too "small potatoes" to upset the established dairy industry, with its sixty-thousand-plus dairy farms accounting for more than $20 billion in annual revenue.[16]

From what I've heard from dairy representatives, though, it's fair to say they don't like the idea of unpasteurized milk, and want to see the regulators crack down hard. At a daylong special symposium on raw milk held in February 2009 by the International Association for Food Protection, a trade organization, a representative of the National Dairy Council, Isabel Maples, justified mandatory pasteurization this way: Milk production, she said, "is not a sterile process. There is certainly the potential for contaminants. Milk is one of the safest, most regulated foods in the American food supply. It is tested up to seventeen times from the cow to the consumer. . . . There are opportunities for contamination, even from healthy cows . . . from milk touching the surface of the cow as she is milked."

In case anyone had any doubts about the need for pasteurization, she fell back on the argument that raw milk opponents frequently fall back on—the fears for the children. "How many of you are parents?" she asked her audience. "When you look at diseases that are possibilities, it's not just stomach illness . . . we're looking at hospitalizations and even death. As parents, we want to provide the best."

From my background writing about small business and entrepreneurship, I always thought one of the big attractions about raw milk is the opportunity for farmers to earn higher margins than they can earn by selling in bulk to large processors. But while a steady and growing stream, on the order of five or more every week, query the Farm-to-Consumer Legal Defense Fund for information on how to set up a herd-share agreement, the dairy industry, in its active opposition to raw milk, has kept the lid on any significant movement by dairy owners to producing raw milk.

This issue came up in stark fashion at the main regulatory industry get-together in April 2009—the biannual meeting of the National Conference of Interstate Milk Shipments. This is the place where regulators examine proposals for changes to the regulations that guide the dairy industry—mainly, the so-called Pasteurized Milk Ordinance, which is the collection of rules and regulations, mainly concerning sanitation, that guide the production and pasteurization of conventional milk in the US.[17]

At that 2009 session, Mark McAfee, owner of Organic Pastures Dairy Co., challenged the regulators to face up to the growth in raw milk consumption by submitting a proposal to lift the federal prohibition on interstate shipments of raw milk. Thinking he'd appeal to the dairy industry's concerns about the feast-or-famine nature of the dairy business, McAfee relied heavily on economics. "I distribute to 400 stores in California," he told a special committee set up to consider proposals relating to raw milk. "I get $150 a hundredweight. Conventional dairies are getting $11 a hundredweight and they are having to cull their herds because they are losing money. We cannot keep the milk on the shelf. There is a reason for this. California consumers enjoy milk that is very safe. It is not the same as the milk intended for pasteurization."

McAfee also spoke about a growing "black market" for raw milk. "I'm here to tell you that's not right." A black market, prompted by the prohibition in many states against selling raw milk, represents more of a safety concern than regulated raw milk, he said.

Only two individuals spoke in active opposition to McAfee's proposals, and both were from the dairy industry. Rob Byrne of the National Milk Producers Federation said he not only was opposed to relaxing the federal ban on interstate milk shipments, but would in fact go farther. "I'd like to see the federal ban extended to include an intrastate ban." In other words, he wants to see the federal government outlaw raw milk entirely.

Jim Howie, with the Southern Marketing Agency, an association of milk producers in the Southeast, ridiculed McAfee for emphasizing the financial benefits he realizes from raw milk. "The Pasteurized Milk Ordinance is a public health document," he said. "This should not be a marketing issue."

He allowed that there is a black market in raw milk. "I cringe when I see it. Authorities need to use the laws·they have to close that black market. If someone gets sick, the newspaper article will not say 'raw milk.' It will say 'milk' . . . and will hurt dairy farmers around the country."

"We have the safest product on the market because of pasteurization. We need to strengthen the laws against raw milk."

When you think about it, the opposition of dairy processors like the Southern Marketing Agency is understandable. In a world where raw milk is more widely available, pasteurized milk sales would inevitably suffer. After all, there really isn't an obvious role for processors when the milk isn't being processed.

No surprise, but the committee hearing McAfee's proposal, consisting of about fifteen regulators, voted unanimously to reject it. A second committee that reviewed all proposals voted similarly.

The openings for compromise seem scant, with the FDA's dairy leadership nearly hysterical in its opposition to raw milk. It sets the tone, since the FDA provides important financial support to state regulators and to the public health community in the form of training and funding of various programs and research. The FDA's regional officials around the country work closely with state officials, and sometimes accompany them on raids of raw dairies.

Indeed, by 2009, it seemed as if the FDA might be girding its loins to push for further limitations on raw milk availability, when Connecticut's Department of Agriculture initiated legislation to ban retail sales of raw milk in that state, which had been allowed for many years. Because Connecticut is so close to New York City and other major population areas, it has been a major supplier to those areas.

Raw milk proponents organized themselves and scuttled the move in committee, producing a number of experts to testify during a day of hearings in February that I attended.[18]

Even when it seemed the legislation was dead, however, the agriculture commissioner, F. Philip Prelli, pushed ahead, trying to get the legislation considered by the entire legislature. As part of that effort, he wrote an opinion piece for the *Hartford Courant* that railed against raw milk.[19]

What struck me about his piece was the suspect evidence he used, as I discussed in this posting on April 5, 2009:

> On the heels of the failure of Connecticut legislation that would have pulled raw milk off the retail shelves in the metropolitan New York City area, a state regulator has come out with what can only be characterized as a tirade against raw milk. And an irresponsible tirade at that.
>
> Here are the two main arguments advanced by F. Philip Prelli, head of Connecticut's Department of Agriculture, and the flaws in his logic:
>
> • **Beware manure.** Prelli's basic argument is that raw milk production involves "a process that inherently is fraught with difficulties because of the high concentration of fecal matter on a dairy farm. . . . Manure will be present where cows are housed and milked." Is he saying something new here? "Fecal matter"—I love his effort to use "scientific" terminology in a subtle effort to generate fear—has been around farms pretty much since the beginning of time, hasn't it? Why should we suddenly be afraid of manure? Because, obviously, he is banking on the fact that many people see themselves as living in a sanitized world, where "fecal matter" doesn't exist.
>
> • **Twisting the data.** Prelli's next argument is that Connecticut has had multiple problems with raw milk. Last summer, he states, "14 people were sickened from consuming unpasteurized milk produced by a Simsbury farm. . . . It was not the first time that illness from consumption of raw milk or raw milk products has occurred in Connecticut." So, I read on, expecting to learn about other cases. If you read closely (and this is part of the data game going on here), you learn

that "in 1990 four cases of campylobacteriosis were linked
to the consumption of raw milk from a Connecticut farm."
That is IT. 18 cases in 18 years—that works out to an average
of ONE illness per year over the previous 18 years.

The rest of Prelli's gibberish—about recalls of raw milk in 2001
and "three occasions over the past five years where action taken by"
ag officials kept bad milk off the market—are irrelevant. No one
became ill, and we know well from experiences in New York and
Pennsylvania that officials frequently find bugs without anyone
becoming ill . . . and then use their findings to generate fear and
congratulate themselves.

That's the bottom line here. Fearmongering. Prelli has presented
a totally bankrupt argument. If raw milk is so dangerous, why even
allow sales from the farm? Why not totally ban it? Actually, that
would probably be the next step in Connecticut if raw milk were
eliminated from retail sales. We'd see a "stepped" approach—get rid
of retail sales first, then move to on-farm sales.

Unfortunately for Prelli and his handlers in Washington, consumers are wising up to the fearmongering, and the Connecticut
restrictions have rightfully been rejected.

Prelli's article reinforces what a big loss the Connecticut legislative initiative was to the FDA and its lackeys within the medical and
food protection communities. They've racked up a couple of big
wins, defeating SB 201 in California and achieving victory against
the Meadowsweet herd share in New York. They obviously don't
take well to losing.[20]

Prelli's article also contained an important message to me. His use of the
data—showing an average of one person per year becoming ill from raw
milk over a period of eighteen years—reaffirmed for me that there's no way
that raw milk can be considered a public health issue. It's a political issue,
pure and simple. Not just an ordinary political issue, but an ideological
issue. The ideology holds that raw milk is unsafe, and so long as a single
person becomes ill, that ideology is affirmed. Of course, there is no arguing
against that ideology (or most ideologies), because in the adherents' eyes,
there really is no way to disprove it.

So where does that leave the future of raw milk? It's hard to be overly optimistic since the federal government, and many state governments, have been nothing less than relentless in their campaign to make raw milk unavailable. They've been at it on and off for nearly a hundred years. No, the regulators are patient people. They keep drawing paychecks regardless of how long it takes.

I was reminded of their persistence in mid-2009, just as editing was being completed on this book. I was put into contact with Max Kane, the founder of a private Wisconsin raw milk club known as Belle's Lunchbox. His club is one of about twenty whose members reside in Illinois. Another club is run by Richard Hebron, the Michigan farmer who was the target of the October 2006 sting operation described in chapter one that helped launch the national campaign against raw milk.

The Wisconsin Department of Agriculture, Trade and Consumer Protection (DATCP) began demanding information from Belle's Lunchbox in late 2008, when a Chicago-area boy who might have drunk raw milk from the club's cows showed some symptoms of brucellosis, a dangerous bovine disease that the Centers for Disease Control says can be passed to humans via consuming raw milk. After extensive testing, the boy was found not to have brucellosis, but that didn't end the matter, as state authorities in late 2008 and early 2009 continued demanding information from Belle's Lunchbox, like its list of members. Max responded with a cease-and-desist order addressed to DATCAP. Two weeks later Kane was served at his home with a subpoena to appear before Wisconsin's Department of Justice and the DATCP to produce documents and answer questions pertaining to him and Belle's Lunchbox.

Suspecting that the FDA was behind the harassment, Max in May 2009 filed a petition in the state requesting ". . . all records, of any and all communications, from January 2005 to present, between DATCP and the FDA, with regards to Max Kane and/or Belle's Lunchbox."

Max is a big proponent of raw milk—during the winter of 2008 he bicycled more than thirty-four hundred miles across the United States (from Virginia to California) as part of a campaign to further its acceptance. During this fifty-day crusade, raw milk made up 85 percent of his diet. He is in the process of developing a film and a book about his cross-country trip.

In June 2009, Max received a package from a DATCP attorney with eight pages of e-mail communication between Wisconsin's DATCP and FDA officials in Chicago.

The e-mails suggested, first, that state officials weren't totally pleased that the boy's tests had come back negative for brucellosis. Robert Ehrenfeldt, administrator of the Division of Animal Health, wrote on December 19, 2008, to several of his state colleagues: "I hope I don't come to resent making this statement but the brucellosis issue may have been the simplest part of this problem and could have been a pretty good lever to use to push the raw milk issue."

But the e-mails also suggested that the regulators had another approach in mind once the brucellosis case fizzled: to go after all twenty Illinois raw milk buyers' clubs. A February 2009 e-mail with the subject "FDA Raw Milk Conference Call" summarized the call from DATCP's perspective. The call had included four DATCP officials, nine FDA officials, two representatives from the Indiana Board of Animal Health, three from the Illinois Department of Public Health, and one from the Michigan Department of Agriculture.

Front and center in their discussions were both Richard Hebron and Mark McAfee, per this summary material:

> Scott McIntire [district director] and Bill Weissinger [Chicago district special assistant] discussed FDA-CHI activities. They have done some Internet searching and identified about 20 milk clubs in Illinois. They prefer to address one person or group at a time and want to start with Richard Hebron, Family Farm Co-op, in Michigan who may be picking milk up at the Hochstettler (sic) Farm in Indiana for delivery in the Chicago area. Hebron has been prosecuted in Michigan for raw milk sales. Hochstettler was sent a warning letter from FDA Detroit for interstate delivery of raw milk.
>
> There was some discussion on where to go from here.
>
> Michelle Svonkin from FDA-OCC [Office of Chief Counsel] gave a short rundown on Organic Pastures prosecution in California.
>
> Larry Stringer [of DATCP] spoke with CFSAN [FDA's Center for Food Safety and Applied Nutrition] about the raw milk issue. They indicated that raw milk sales are a high priority to them as a significant health risk.

This strategy session shows clearly the preference of the FDA and state agencies to target one raw milk producer or distributor at a time, presumably to send a message to deter others from thinking such foolishness. And the focus on Richard Hebron because he was previously "prosecuted" is curious. He was never prosecuted, never even went before a judge. But apparently, because he was targeted by Michigan authorities for an ill-considered sting operation, he's now akin to an ex-felon—a target that's easy to justify to the public because, after all, authorities went after him once before in a big way. And the federal prosecution of Organic Pastures has become a neat template for others that may well follow.

In my view, given the likely continuing government offensive, the main hopes for raw milk advocates lie in the following trends:

- **An organized and active group of consumers fighting on behalf of the right to obtain raw milk and nutrient-dense foods in general.** It was a coalition of consumers that beat back Commissioner Prelli in Connecticut, and the movement is spreading. Coalitions of consumers have sprung up to push raw milk legislation not only in Connecticut but also in Maryland, Ohio, Pennsylvania, and, of course, California. One umbrella organization is the National Independent Consumers and Farmers Association.
- **More impartial reporting on raw milk by the media.** As I recounted in chapter 1, media reports about events like the sting operation against Richard Hebron in Michigan or the abusive questioning of Gary Oaks in a Cincinnati parking lot tended to emphasize the regulator viewpoint. Since 2006, the media have gradually become more accepting of the raw milk consumer position, such as in a major *New York Times* article on the growing popularity of raw milk.[21] By 2009, the Food Network had even done a highly favorable televised segment on raw milk.
- **An ever-growing consumer demand for raw milk,** which entices increasing numbers of farmers to take the risk, and seek out the potentially higher profits that go with producing and distributing raw milk.
- **A growing black market.** I've refrained from saying much about this, in line with my commitment not to get farmers into trouble. But I know of many farmers supplying raw milk illegally to consumers and to medical personnel, who sell it to their patients. An article at msn.com about "Trafficking in Raw Milk" said, "After illegal drugs, raw milk . . . may be the most briskly traded underground commodity in America."[22]
- **Growing concern about the rapid increases in chronic disease rates,** and a realization that our health care system is geared toward

alleviating symptoms and not exploring the power of nutrition for heading off illness. The emergence of the international Slow Food (as opposed to fast food) movement, along with the growing demand for locally produced and organic foods, exemplifies this shift in public perception.

Trying to be realistic, I would say the fight over raw milk could go either way. I like to be optimistic, though, and I believe that Americans' natural inclination toward independence and openness to new ideas makes it tough for the bureaucrats to win in the long run against a determined populace. One thing is for sure: If secretive government regulators are successful in their efforts to deprive consumers of unpasteurized dairy products, they will be emboldened to push us farther toward their vision of reliance on sterile factory food. The only choice, at that point, will be to own your own cow, and—who knows?—they might just figure out ways to keep owners from consuming that milk as well.

ENDNOTES

Introduction: Why Raw Milk So Inflames the Passions

1. MacDonald, James M., et al. "Changes in the Size and Location of US Dairy Farms" (chapter from USDA report "Profits, Costs, and the Changing Structure of Dairy Farming/ERR-47") (September 2007). Available online at www.ers.usda.gov/publications/err47/err47b.pdf. Accessed May 3, 2009.
2. Ibid.
3. Testimony of Pennsylvania Department of Agriculture Secretary Dennis C. Wolff at Raw Milk Hearing, September 18, 2007. Available online at http://senatorbrubaker.com/agriculture/091807/Wolff2.pdf. Accessed July 2, 2009.
4. Hoppe, Robert A., et al. "Structure and Finances of US Farms: Family Farm Report, 2007 Edition." *Economic Information Bulletin* EIB-24 (June 2007). Available online at www.ers.usda.gov/publications/eib24/eib24b.pdf. Accessed May 3, 2009.
5. www.thecompletepatient.com/journal/2007/4/22/resistance-tales-updates-on-nais-nutritionist-registration-and-raw-milk.html#comments. Accessed May 3, 2009.
6. Jarvis, William T. "Raw Milk Can Be Deadly" (1997). Available online at www.ncahf.org/articles/o-r/rawmilk.html. Accessed May 3, 2009.
7. Barrett, Stephen. "Why Raw Milk Should Be Avoided" (December 22, 2003). Available online at www.quackwatch.com/01QuackeryRelatedTopics/rawmilk.html. Accessed May 3, 2009.
8. www.thecompletepatient.com/journal/2008/12/11/how-does-the-president-elect-feel-about-raw-milk-lets-say-he.html. Accessed May 3, 2009.
9. www.nicfa.com/stateassociations.html. Accessed July 2, 2009.

Chapter 1: Why Is the Government Kicking Around a Bunch of Small Dairy Farmers?

1. www.fda.gov. Accessed March 12, 2009.
2. www.deecreekfarm.com. Accessed March 12, 2009.
3. Gumpert, David. "A Federal Blight for Cherry Farmers." *BusinessWeek* (June 27, 2006). Available online at www.businessweek.com/smallbiz/content/jun2006/sb20060626_541703.htm?chan=search. Accessed March 12, 2009.
4. www.organicpastures.com, Accessed June 13, 2009
5. Gumpert, David. "Getting a Raw Deal?" *BusinessWeek* (September 28, 2006). Available online at www.businessweek.com/smallbiz/content/sep2006/sb20060928_865207.htm?chan=search. Accessed March 12, 2009.
6. www.thecompletepatient.com. Accessed March 12, 2009.

7. Gumpert, David. "States Target Raw-Milk Farmers." *BusinessWeek* (October 19, 2006). Available online at www.businessweek.com/smallbiz/content/oct2006/ sb20061019_952010.htm. Accessed March 12, 2009.

8. "Kentucky Man Guilty in Ohio Milk Sale." *Farm and Dairy* (November 23, 2006). Available online at www.farmanddairy.com/news/kentucky-man-guilty-in-ohio-raw-milk-sale/3650.html. Accessed June 30, 2009.

Chapter 2: Raw Milk and the Upside-Down World of Food-Borne Illness

1. Porter, Charles Sanford. *Milk Diet: As a Remedy for Chronic Disease*. West Bend, Wisconsin: God's Whey, LLC, 2005 (copyright Century Types).

2. Tauxe, Robert V. "Food Safety and Irradiation: Protecting the Public from Foodborne Infections." *Emerging Infectious Diseases* 7.3 supplement (2001): 516–521. Available online at www.cdc.gov/ncidod/eid/vol7no3_supp/tauxe.htm. Accessed March 14, 2009.

3. Wells, J. G., et al. "Laboratory Investigation of Hemorrhagic Colitis Outbreaks Associated with a Rare *Escherichia coli* Serotype." *Journal of Clinical Microbiology* 18.3 (1983): 512–520. Available online at http://www.pubmedcentral.nih.gov/ articlerender.fcgi?artid=270845. Accessed March 14, 2009.

4. www.westonaprice.org. Accessed March 14, 2009.

5. www.thecompletepatient.com/journal/2006/10/26/michigan-whodunit-guess-what-caused-illness-that-sparked-mas.html. Accessed June 30, 2009.

6. Wong, C. S., et al. "The Risk of the Hemolytic-Uremic Syndrome After Antibiotic Treatment of *Escherichia coli* O157:H7." *New England Journal of Medicine* 342.26 (2000): 1930–1936. Available online at http://content.nejm.org/cgi/content/ full/342/26/1930. Accessed March 15, 2009.

7. Allen, Nancy. "Darke County Farm Can Still Sell Milk." Celina, Ohio, *Daily Standard* (October 10, 2006). Available online at www.dailystandard.com/date/2006/10/10/ news/headline1.htm. Accessed March 14, 2009.

Chapter 3: Why Are We Still Debating Pasteurization?

1. www.thecompletepatient.com/journal/2007/7/28/from-the-latest-ny-raw-milk-listeria-target-we-worked-too-ha.html. Accessed March 14, 2009.

2. http://en.wikipedia.org/wiki/Pasteurization. Accessed March 14, 2009.

3. www.thecompletepatient.com/journal/2007/8/16/to-the-fda-question-of-raw-milk-safety-and-availability-is-n.html. Accessed March 14, 2009.

4. www.cfsan.fda.gov/~dms/rawmilk2/sld030.htm. Accessed March 14, 2009.

5. www.thecompletepatient.com/journal/2007/4/2/memoir-of-a-raw-milk-illness-turned-medical-nightmare-part-2.html. Accessed March 14, 2009.

6. www.thecompletepatient.com/journal/2007/4/2/memoir-of-a-raw-milk-illness-turned-medical-nightmare-part-2.html?currentPage=2#comments. Accessed March 14, 2009.

7. Schmid, Ron. *The Untold Story of Milk*. Winona Lake, Indiana: New Trends Publishing, 2003.

8. Hartley, Robert. *An Historical, Scientific, and Practical Essay on Milk as an Article of Human Sustenance*. Manchester, New Hampshire: Ayer Publishing, 1977. Available online at http://books.google.com/books?id=i1p3WSCex0EC&pg=PA132&lpg=PA 132&dq=Robert+Hartley,+distillery+dairies&source=bl&ots=0CRTmdjcw0&sig=8 zzBeAxsvXT09OmyldvAPvpezk&hl=en&ei=DjOxSZfoENLjtgf8tKzCBw&sa=X&oi =book_result&resnum=7&ct=result#PPA139,M1. Accessed March 14, 2009.

9. Ibid., p. 174.

10. Debré, Patrice. *Louis Pasteur*. Baltimore, Maryland: Johns Hopkins University Press, 1998, pp. 235–238.

11. Reynolds, Moira Davidson. *How Pasteur Changed History: The Story of Louis Pasteur and the Pasteur Institute*. Sarasota, Florida: McGuinn & McGuire Publishing, 1994, p. 36.

12. Ibid., pp. 41–42.

13. Schmid, p. 44.

14. Debré, p. 359.

15. Ibid., p. 360.

16. http://en.wikipedia.org/wiki/Ilya_Ilyich_Mechnikov. Accessed March 14, 2009.

17. Czaplicki, Alan. "Pure Milk Is Better than Purified Milk." *Social Science History* 31.3 (2007): 411–433. Available online at http://ssh.dukejournals.org/cgi/ reprint/31/3/411. Accessed March 14, 2009.

18. Crewe, J. R. "Real Milk Cures Many Diseases." Originally published in *Certified Milk Magazine* (January 1929). Available online at www.realmilk.com/milkcure.html. Accessed March 14, 2009.

19. Tauxe, Robert V. "Food Safety and Irradiation: Protecting the Public from Foodborne Infections." *Emerging Infectious Diseases* 7.3 supplement (2001): 516–521. Available online at www.cdc.gov/ncidod/eid/vol7no3_supp/tauxe.htm. Accessed March 15, 2009.

20. Schmid, pp. 54–55.

21. www.thecompletepatient.com/journal/2007/9/22/gold-in-them-thar-raw-milk-tanks-seeking-justice-in-the-righ.html#comment1013120. Accessed March 15, 2009.

22. Wells, J. G., et al. "Laboratory Investigation of Hemorrhagic Colitis Outbreaks Associated with a Rare *Escherichia coli* Serotype." *Journal of Clinical Microbiology* 18.3 (1983): 512–520. Available online at http://jcm.asm.org/cgi/reprint/18/3/512?vi ew=long&pmid=6355145. Accessed March 15, 2009.

23. Klevens, R. M., et al. "Invasive Methicillin-Resistant *Staphylococcus aureus* Infections in the United States." *Journal of the American Medical Association* 298.15 (2007): 1763–1771. Available online at http://jama.ama-assn.org/cgi/content/ full/298/15/1763. Accessed March 15, 2009.

24. Levy, Stuart B. "Antibacterial Household Products: Cause for Concern." *Emerging Infectious Diseases* 7.3 supplement (2001): 512–515. Available online at www.cdc .gov/ncidod/eid/vol7no3_supp/levy.htm. Accessed March 15, 2009.
25. www.organicpastures.com/faq.html. Accessed March 15, 2009.

Chapter 4: Picking Up the Pieces

1. Michigan Department of Agriculture. *Dairy Digest* (Summer 2002). Available online at www.michigan.gov/documents/MDA_FDD_Dairy_Digest_ Summer_2002_42473_7.pdf. Accessed March 21, 2009.
2. Michigan Public Acts of 2000, No. 92. *Food Law of 2000*. Available online at www.legislature.mi.gov/(S(j5sznx45si354k45vyfeh055))/mileg.aspx?page=getobject &objectname=mcl-act-92-of-2000&queryid=860762&highlight=. Accessed March 21, 2009.
3. *Schmitmeyer v. Ohio Department of Agriculture,* Case No. 06-CV-63277, Darke County Court of Common Pleas (Ohio), December 29, 2006. Available online at www.davidgumpert.com/files/12_29_06_decisi.pdf. Accessed March 21, 2009.
4. Testimony of Stephen Beam from Deposition, April 7, 2008, in case *Organic Pastures Dairy Company, LLC, and Claravale Farm, Inc. v. State of California and A. G. Kawamura, Secretary of California Department of Food and Agriculture,* Case No. CU-07-00204, Superior Court of San Benito County (California).

Chapter 5: Raw Milk and the Cases of the Disappearing Pathogens

1. Gumpert, David. "The Investigative Farmer." *BusinessWeek* (July 11, 2007). Available online at www.businessweek.com/smallbiz/content/jul2007/sb20070711_965352_ page_2.htm. Accessed March 21, 2009.
2. www.thecompletepatient.com/journal/2007/7/28/from-the-latest-ny-raw-milk-listeria-target-we-worked-too-ha.html. Accessed March 21, 2009.
3. California Department of Food and Agriculture. "Listeria Detected in Organic Pastures Raw Cream." Press release (September 7, 2007). Available online at www .cdfa.ca.gov/egov/Press_Releases/Press_Release.asp?PRnum=07-068. Accessed March 21, 2009.
4. www.thecompletepatient.com/journal/nearly-a-year-to-the-day-after-shutdown-the-raw-milk-inspect.html#comment986043. Accessed March 22, 2009.
5. New York State Department of Agriculture and Markets. "Autumn Valley Farm Voluntarily Suspends Direct Sale of Raw Milk to Consumers." Press release (August 1, 2008). Available online at www.agmkt.state.ny.us/AD/alert.asp?ReleaseID=843. Accessed March 22, 2009.
6. www.thecompletepatient.com/journal/2008/8/5/caught-in-the-act-lori-and-darren-mcgrath-gain-support-for-a.html#comments. Accessed March 22, 2009.

7. Hitchins, A. D., and R. C. Whiting. "Food-Borne *Listeria monocytogenes* Risk Assessment." *Food Additives and Contaminants* 18.12 (2001): 1108–1117(10). Available online at www.ingentaconnect.com/content/tandf/tfac/2001/00000018/00000012/art00008. Accessed March 22, 2009.

8. Chen, Yuhuan, et al. "*Listeria monocytogenes*: Low Levels Equal Low Risk." *Journal of Food Protection* 66.4 (2003): 570–577. Available online at http://apt.allenpress.com/perlserv/?request=get-abstract&doi=10.1043%2F0362-028X(2003)066[0570%3AMLLELR]2.3.CO%3B2&ct=1. Accessed March 22, 2009.

9. US Food and Drug Administration and US Food Safety and Inspection Service. "FDA, FSIS Statement on CDC Listeria Study." Press release (April 14, 1992). Available online at www.fda.gov/bbs/topics/ANSWERS/ANS00393.html. Accessed March 22, 2009.

10. US Food and Drug Administration and US Food Safety and Inspection Service. "Draft Assessment of the Relative Risk to Public Health from Foodborne *Listeria monocytogenes* Among Selected Categories of Ready-to-Eat Foods" (January 2001). Available online at www.foodsafety.gov/~dms/lmriskex.html. Accessed March 22, 2009.

11. www.thecompletepatient.com/journal/2009/2/12/chuck-phippens-germ-war-with-ny-ag-markets-how-many-listeria.html. Accessed March 22, 2009.

12. www.thecompletepatient.com/journal/2009/6/6/ny-ag-officials-make-clear-their-position-on-listeria-is-usd.html. Accessed July 1, 2009.

13. www.thecompletepatient.com/journal/2008/8/5/caught-in-the-act-lori-and-darren-mcgrath-gain-support-for-a.html?currentPage=2#comments. Accessed March 22, 2009.

Chapter 6: What Are We to Make of So Much Anecdotal Evidence?

1. www.thecompletepatient.com/journal/2007/3/22/what-do-you-do-when-a-neighbor-wants-some-of-your-raw-milk-for-her-child.html#comments. Accessed April 7, 2009.

2. www.westonaprice.org/children/dietformothers.html. Accessed April 7, 2009.

3. US Food and Drug Administration's Center for Food Safety and Applied Nutrition. "The Dangers of Raw Milk: Unpasteurized Milk Can Pose a Serious Health Risk." FOODFACTS series (October 2006). Available online at www.cfsan.fda.gov/~dms/rawmilk.html. Accessed April 7, 2009.

4. www.thecompletepatient.com/journal/2009/1/21/the-regulators-would-prefer-us-to-be-divided-so-they-can-con.html. Accessed April 7, 2009.

5. www.youtube.com/watch?v=xudsY0E0bVI. Accessed April 7, 2009.

6. Bradley, John, Larry K. Pickering, and John Jareb. "Advise Families Against Giving Children Raw Milk." *AAP News* 29.12 (2008). Available online at www.marlerblog.com/uploads/file/JPedArticle.pdf. Accessed April 7, 2009.

7. www.thecompletepatient.com/journal/2007/3/24/the-nuances-of-educating-people-about-raw-milk-and-other-real-foods.html#comments. Accessed April 7, 2009.

8. www.thecompletepatient.com/journal/2008/12/14/finally-a-way-to-excite-the-regulators-a-las-vegas-dad-pours.html#comments. Accessed April 7, 2009.

Chapter 7: Is Raw Milk Really Healthier?

1. US Food and Drug Administration. "Problems Digesting Dairy Products?" FDA Consumer Health Information Update series (2009). Available online at www.fda .gov/consumer/updates/lactose032508.html. Accessed April 13, 2009.

2. Akinbami, Lara J. "The State of Childhood Asthma, United States, 1980–2005." *Advance Data from Vital and Health Statistics* 381 (2006). National Center for Health Statistics. Available online at www.cdc.gov/nchs/data/ad/ad381.pdf. Accessed April 13, 2009.

3. "Causes of Adult Asthma" (2006). Available online at www.healthcentral.com/asthma/introduction-000004_3-145.html?ic=4004. Accessed April 13, 2009.

4. Kalb, Claudia. "Fear and Allergies in the Classroom." *Newsweek* (November 5, 2007). Available online at www.newsweek.com/id/62296/page/2. Accessed April 13, 2009.

5. "What's in Raw Milk?" (2009). Available online at www.raw-milk-facts.com/what_is_in_raw_milk.html. Accessed April 13, 2009.

6. Schmid, Ron. *The Untold Story of Milk*. Winona Lake, Indiana: New Trends Publishing, 2003, p. 232.

7. www.thecompletepatient.com/journal/2008/2/23/at-last-data-on-raw-milk-and-lactose-intolerance-raw-milk-le.html. Accessed April 13, 2009.

8. US Food and Drug Administration. "Problems Digesting Dairy Products?" FDA Consumer Health Information Update series (2009). Available online at www.fda .gov/consumer/updates/lactose032508.html. Accessed April 13, 2009.

9. Sheehan, John F. "On the Safety of Raw Milk (With a Word About Pasteurization)." Slide 13 of 69 of slide-show presentation (May 12, 2005). Available online at www.cfsan.fda.gov/~ear/milksafe/milksa13.htm. Accessed April 14, 2009.

10. Ibid., slide 47.

11. Weston A. Price Foundation. "Response to the FDA: A Point-by-Point Rebuttal to the Anti-Raw Milk PowerPoint Presentation by John F. Sheehan, BSc (Dy), JD, Division of Dairy and Egg Safety" (2007). Available online at www.realmilk.com/documents/SheehanPowerPointResponse.pdf. Accessed April 13, 2009.

12. Ibid.

13. Sheehan, slide 60.

14. Ibid., slide 65.

15. http://en.wikipedia.org/wiki/Ilya_Ilyich_Mechnikov. Accessed April 13, 2009.

16. http://en.wikipedia.org/wiki/Probiotic. Accessed April 13, 2009.

17. Ibid.

18. Hatakka, K., et al. "Effect of Long Term Consumption of Probiotic Milk on Infections in Children Attending Day Care Centres: Double Blind, Randomised Trial." *British Medical Journal* 322.7298 (2001): 1327. Available online at www.bmj .com/cgi/content/full/322/7298/1327. Accessed April 13, 2009.

19. Wen, Li, et al. "Innate Immunity and Intestinal Microbiota in the Development of Type 1 Diabetes." *Nature* 455 (2008): 1109–1113.Available online at www .nature.com/nature/journal/v455/n7216/full/nature07336.html. Accessed July 1, 2009. Summary available online at www.shvoong.com/medicine-and-health/ epidemiology-public-health/1840833-good-gut-bacteria-protect-diabetes. Accessed July 1, 2009.

20. www.danactive.com/danactive_how.html. Accessed April 13, 2009.

21. www.thecompletepatient.com/journal/2008/12/11/how-does-the-president-elect-feel-about-raw-milk-lets-say-he.html#comments. Accessed April 13, 2009.

22. Waser, M., et al. "Inverse Association of Farm Milk Consumption with Asthma and Allergy in Rural and Suburban Populations Across Europe." *Clinical and Experimental Allergy* 37.5 (2007): 661–670. Available online at www3.interscience .wiley.com/journal/117999972/abstract. Accessed April 13, 2009.

23. Perkin, M. R. "Unpasteurized Milk: Health or Hazard?" *Clinical and Experimental Allergy* 37.5 (2007): 627–630. Available online at www3.interscience.wiley.com/ journal/117999990/abstract. Accessed April 13, 2009.

24. Asthma and Allergy Foundation of America. "Asthma Facts and Figures." www.aafa .org/display.cfm?id=8&sub=42. Accessed April 13, 2009.

25. Perkin.

26. Bernstein, Henry. "Dangers of Consuming Raw Milk: Reasons for Thinking Twice Before Consuming Unpasteurized Dairy Products." Harvard Health Publications series (2009). Available online at http://health.msn.com/kids-health/articlepage .aspx?cp-documentid=100220425&GT1=3103. Accessed April 13, 2009.

27. Bradley, John, Larry K. Pickering, and John Jareb. "Advise Families Against Giving Children Raw Milk." *AAP News* 29.12 (2008). Available online at www.marlerblog .com/uploads/file/JPedArticle.pdf. Accessed April 13, 2009.

28. Lejeune, Jeffrey T., and Päivi J. Rajala-Schultz. "Unpasteurized Milk: A Continued Public Health Threat." *Clinical Infectious Diseases* 48.S1 (2009): 93–100. Available online at www.thecompletepatient.com/storage/InfectDis-Anti1-09.pdf. Accessed April 13, 2009.

29. Marler, Bill. "Raw Milk Pros: Review of the Peer-Reviewed Literature." Editorial (June 6, 2008). Available online at www.marlerblog.com/2008/06/articles/lawyer-oped/raw-milk-pros-review-of-the-peerreviewed-literature. Accessed April 13, 2009.

Chapter 8: How Dangerous Is Raw Milk, Really?

1. www.ftcldf.org. Accessed April 18, 2009.

2. Fleming, David W., et al. "Pasteurized Milk as a Vehicle of Infection in an Outbreak of Listeriosis." *New England Journal of Medicine* 312.7 (1985): 404–407. Available online at http://content.nejm.org/cgi/content/abstract/312/7/404. Accessed April 18, 2009.

3. Ryan, C. A., et al. "Massive Outbreak of Antimicrobial-Resistant Salmonellosis Traced to Pasteurized Milk." *Journal of the American Medical Association* 258.22 (1987): 3269–3274. Available online at www.ncbi.nlm.nih.gov/ pubmed/3316720?dopt=Abstract. Accessed April 18, 2009.

4. Hennessy, T. W., et al. "A National Outbreak of *Salmonella enteritidis* Infections from Ice Cream." *New England Journal of Medicine* 334.20 (1996): 1281–1286. Available online at www.ncbi.nlm.nih.gov/pubmed/8609944. Accessed April 18, 2009.

5. Thompson, Don. "Spoiled Milk Apparently Sickened 1,300 Inmates at 11 Prisons." Associated Press (June 2, 2006). Available online at www.campylobacterblog .com/2006/06/articles/campylobacter-watch/spoiled-milk-apparently-sickened- 1300-inmates-at-11-prisons. Accessed April 18, 2009.

6. Sheehan, John F. "On the Safety of Raw Milk (With a Word About Pasteurization)." Slide-show presentation (May 12, 2005). Available online at www.cfsan.fda .gov/~ear/milksafe/milksafe.htm. Accessed April 18, 2009.

7. Ibid., slide 67.

8. Weston A. Price Foundation. "Response to the FDA: A Point-by-Point Rebuttal to the Anti-Raw Milk PowerPoint Presentation by John F. Sheehan, BSc (Dy), JD, Division of Dairy and Egg Safety" (2007). Available online at www.realmilk.com/ documents/SheehanPowerPointResponse.pdf. Accessed April 18, 2009.

9. Sheehan, slide 14.

10. Weston A. Price Foundation, p. 14.

11. Van Kessel, J. S., et al. "Prevalence of Salmonellae, *Listeria monocytogenes,* and Fecal Coliforms in Bulk Tank Milk on US Dairies." *Journal of Dairy Science* 87 (2004): 2822–2830. Available online at http://jds.fass.org/cgi/content/full/87/9/2822?gca=87 %2F9%2F2822&sendit=Get+All+Checked+Abstract(s)&. Accessed April 18, 2009.

12. Sheehan, slide 22.

13. Weston A. Price Foundation, p. 22.

14. Sheehan, slide 26.

15. Weston A. Price Foundation, p. 26.

16. Headrick, Marcia L., et al. "The Epidemiology of Raw Milk–Associated Foodborne Disease Outbreaks Reported in the United States, 1973 through 1992." *American Journal of Public Health* 88.8 (1998): 1219–1221. Available online at www.ajph.org/ cgi/reprint/88/8/1219. Accessed April 18, 2009.

17. Smith DeWaal, Caroline. "Raw Milk Consumption: A Consumer Viewpoint." Presentation at International Association for Food Protection's Symposium "Raw Milk Consumption: An Emerging Public Health Threat?" Arlington, Virginia (February 17, 2009). Available online at www.foodprotection.org/files/timely- topics/TT_04.pdf. Accessed April 18, 2009.

18. Langer, Adam J. "Do State Raw Milk Sales Restrictions Reduce Raw Milk Outbreaks?: A Policy Analysis." Presentation at International Association for Food Protection's Symposium "Raw Milk Consumption: An Emerging Public Health Threat?" Arlington, Virginia (February 17, 2009). Available online at www .foodprotection.org/files/timely-topics/TT_07.pdf. Accessed April 18, 2009.

19. www.thecompletepatient.com/journal/2007/3/29/chewing-on-a-mothers-real-message-about-raw-milk-and-the-risks-of-dramatic-stories.html ?currentPage=2#comments. Accessed April 18, 2009.

20. Sofos, John N. "*Listeria monocytogenes* and Listeriosis." Slide-show presentation. Available online at www.fsis.usda.gov/PDF/Slides_092806_JSofos.pdf. Accessed April 18, 2009.

21. Centers for Disease Control and Prevention. *Foodborne Diseases Active Surveillance Network (FoodNet): Population Survey Atlas of Exposures, 2002.* Atlanta: Centers for Disease Control and Prevention, 2004, pp. 204–205.

22. Fallon, Sally. "*E. coli* O157:H7 Outbreak in Washington State: Lessons Learned" (2006). Available online at www.realmilk.com/washington-lessons-learned.html. Accessed April 18, 2009.

23. www.thecompletepatient.com/journal/2009/4/3/can-pathogens-survive-in-grass-fed-raw-milk-an-old-debate-ke.html. Accessed April 18, 2009.

24. Blaser, M. J., E. Sazie, and L. P. Williams Jr. "The Influence of Immunity on Raw Milk–Associated Campylobacter Infection." *Journal of the American Medical Association* 257.1 (1987): 43–46. Available online at http://jama.ama-assn.org/cgi/content/abstract/257/1/43?maxtoshow=&HITS=10&hits=10&RESULTFORMAT=&fulltext=blaser%2C+sazie&searchid=1&FIRSTINDEX=0&resourcetype=HWCIT. Accessed April 18, 2009.

25. www.thecompletepatient.com/journal/2009/4/6/sore-loser-did-the-fda-ghost-write-the-connecticut-ag-chiefs.html?currentPage=3#comments. Accessed April 18, 2009.

26. www.thecompletepatient.com/journal/2009/4/12/a-colorado-dairy-owner-on-the-hot-seat-shares-his-sense-of-r.html?currentPage=1#comments. Accessed April 18, 2009.

Chapter 9: *E. coli* O157:H7 and the Education of Mary McGonigle-Martin

1. Centers for Disease Control and Prevention. "Foodborne Illness, Technical Information" (2005). Available online at www.cdc.gov/ncidod/dbmd/diseaseinfo/foodborneinfections_t.htm. Accessed April 18, 2009.

2. Here is one example of a public health questionnaire, a Massachusetts Department of Public Health Foodborne Illness Complaint Worksheet: www.mass.gov/Eeohhs2/docs/dph/environmental/foodsafety/foodborne_ill_worksheet.doc. Accessed April 19, 2009.

3. Smith DeWaal, Caroline. "Raw Milk Consumption: A Consumer Viewpoint." Presentation at International Association for Food Protection's Symposium "Raw Milk Consumption: An Emerging Public Health Threat?" Arlington, Virginia (February 17, 2009). Available online at www.foodprotection.org/files/timely-topics/TT_04.pdf. Accessed April 19, 2009.

4. Jay, Michele T., et al. "*Escherichia coli* O157:H7 in Feral Swine Near Spinach Fields and Cattle, Central California Coast." *Emerging Infectious Diseases* 13.12 (2007).

Available online at www.cdc.gov/eid/content/13/12/1908.htm. Accessed April 19, 2009.

5. Schmid, Ron. *The Untold Story of Milk,* revised and updated. Winona Lake, Indiana: New Trends Publishing, 2009, p. 318.

6. California Food Emergency Response Team. *Investigation of an Escherichia coli O157:H7 Outbreak Associated with Dole Pre-Packaged Spinach.* Sacramento: California Department of Health Services, 2007. Available online at www.dhs .ca.gov/fdb/local/PDF/2006%20Spinach%20Report%20Final%20redacted.PDF. Accessed April 19, 2009.

7. CNN Special Investigations Unit. "Danger: Poisoned Food." Aired July 5, 2008. Transcript available online at http://transcripts.cnn.com/TRANSCRIPTS/0807/05/ siu.01.html. Accessed April 19, 2009.

8. California Department of Health Services. "CA-EPI 06-06: *Escherichia coli* O157:H7 Infections in Children Associated with Raw Milk" (February 6, 2007). Available online at www.marlerblog.com/uploads/file/OP%20SDL%20Attachments%20 2%20CDHS%20Final%20Report.pdf. Accessed April 19, 2009.

9. www.realmilk.com/update-ca.html. Accessed April 19, 2009.

10. www.thecompletepatient.com/journal/2007/3/29/chewing-on-a-mothers-real-message-about-raw-milk-and-the-risks-of-dramatic-stories.html#comments. Accessed April 19, 2009.

11. www.thecompletepatient.com/journal/2007/4/5/thoughts-on-raw-milk-and-belief-systems.html#comments. Accessed April 19, 2009.

12. www.thecompletepatient.com/journal/2007/3/29/chewing-on-a-mothers-real-message-about-raw-milk-and-the-risks-of-dramatic-stories.html#comments. Accessed April 19, 2009.

13. Ibid.

14. www.thecompletepatient.com/journal/2007/4/22/resistance-tales-updates-on-nais-nutritionist-registration-and-raw-milk.html#comments. Accessed April 19, 2009.

15. Ibid.

16. Ibid.

17. Ibid.

18. www.thecompletepatient.com/journal/2007/4/22/resistance-tales-updates-on-nais-nutritionist-registration-and-raw-milk.html?currentPage=4#comments. Accessed April 19, 2009.

19. www.thecompletepatient.com/journal/2007/4/22/resistance-tales-updates-on-nais-nutritionist-registration-and-raw-milk.html?currentPage=2#comments. Accessed April 19, 2009.

20. www.thecompletepatient.com/journal/mark-mcafee-on-charges-he-changes-his-story-whats-the-point.html. Accessed April 19, 2009.

21. www.thecompletepatient.com/journal/mark-mcafee-on-charges-he-changes-his-story-whats-the-point.html#comments. Accessed April 19, 2009.

22. www.thecompletepatient.com/journal/nearly-a-year-to-the-day-after-shutdown-the-raw-milk-inspect.html#comments. Accessed April 19, 2009.

23. California Department of Health Services. "CA-EPI 06-06: *Escherichia coli* O157:H7 Infections in Children Associated with Raw Milk" (February 6, 2007). Available

online at www.marlerblog.com/uploads/file/OP%20SDL%20Attachments%20 2%20CDHS%20Final%20Report.pdf. Accessed April 19, 2009.

24. www.thecompletepatient.com/journal/2008/2/9/will-a-court-suit-help-produce-truth-and-justice-in-the-ca-c.html. Accessed April 19, 2009.

25. www.rebuild-from-depression.com/blog/2008/04/the_elephant_in_the_raw_milk_r.html. Accessed April 19, 2009.

26. www.rebuild-from-depression.com/blog/2008/04/the_elephant_in_the_raw_milk_r.html#comments. Accessed April 19, 2009.

27. www.thecompletepatient.com/journal/2008/2/9/will-a-court-suit-help-produce-truth-and-justice-in-the-ca-c.html#comments. Accessed April 19, 2009.

28. www.marlerblog.com/2009/03/articles/lawyer-oped/obama-on-food-safety-this-is-why-what-you-do-is-so-important. Accessed April 19, 2009.

29. Marler, Bill. "Organic Pastures *E. coli* O157:H7 2006 Outbreak" (2009). Available online at www.marlerblog.com/uploads/file/Organic%20Pastures%202006%20 Outbreak.pdf. Accessed April 19, 2009.

30. www.marlerblog.com/2009/03/articles/lawyer-oped/organic-pastures-dairy-e-coli-o157h7-raw-milk-product-outbreak-2006. Accessed July 1, 2009.

31. Marler, p. 6.

32. Ibid., p. 8.

33. Ibid., p. 11.

34. Weston A. Price Foundation. "California Government Official Lies About Raw Milk." Press release (January 4, 2008). Available online at www.westonaprice.org/federalupdate/aa2008/04jan08.html. Accessed April 19, 2009.

Chapter 10: When It Comes to Food, How Much Freedom Should We Have to Take Risks?

1. www.thecompletepatient.com/journal/2007/4/24/is-that-all-there-is-michigan-department-of-agriculture-quietly-settles-with-richard-hebron-in-raw-milk-case .html. Accessed April 19, 2009.

2. Farm-to-Consumer Legal Defense Fund. "Learn More—Cow and Goat-Shares." Available online at www.ftcldf.org/cow-shares.html. Accessed April 19, 2009.

3. MacDonald, James M., et al. "Changes in the Size and Location of US Dairy Farms" (chapter from USDA report "Profits, Costs, and the Changing Structure of Dairy Farming/ERR-47") (September 2007). Available online at www.ers.usda.gov/publications/err47/err47b.pdf. Accessed July 2, 2009.

4. Farm-to-Consumer Legal Defense Fund. "Learn More—Cow and Goat-Shares." Available online at www.ftcldf.org/cow-shares.html. Accessed April 19, 2009.

5. www.thecompletepatient.com/journal/2008/4/8/confessions-of-a-raw-milk-undercover-agent-behind-the-scenes.html#comments. Accessed April 19, 2009.

6. www.thecompletepatient.com/journal/2008/5/6/at-mark-nolt-trial-a-hint-of-hesitation-from-a-bureaucrat-en.html#comments. Accessed April 19, 2009.

7. www.thecompletepatient.com/journal/2008/5/7/a-victory-for-raw-dairy-farmer-glen-wise-as-the-pdas-legal-m.html. Accessed April 19, 2009.

8. www.thecompletepatient.com/journal/2007/12/21/search-warrant-struggle-the-cat-and-mouse-game-between-smith.html. Accessed April 19, 2009.

9. www.thecompletepatient.com/journal/2007/12/21/search-warrant-struggle-the-cat-and-mouse-game-between-smith.html#comments. Accessed April 19, 2009.

Chapter 11: Nine Words Ignite a Raw Milk Battle, California-Style

1. California Assembly Bill No. 1735 (2007). *Milk and Dairy Products: Standards.* Available online at www.leginfo.ca.gov/pub/07-08/bill/asm/ab_1701-1750/ab_1735_bill_20071008_chaptered.html. Accessed May 2, 2009.

2. www.thecompletepatient.com/journal/2007/9/27/a-peek-into-the-future-of-raw-milk-the-worlds-biggest-cowsha.html. Accessed May 2, 2009.

3. Schmid, Ron. "The Vendetta Against Alta Dena Dairy" (2003). Available online at www.realmilk.com/untoldstory_2.html. Accessed May 2, 2009.

4. Ibid.

5. Jarvis, William T. "Raw Milk Can Be Deadly" (1997). Available online at www.ncahf.org/articles/o-r/rawmilk.html. Accessed May 2, 2009.

6. Respondents' Brief in *Organic Pastures Dairy Company, LLC and Claravale Farm, Inc. v. State of California and A. G. Kawamura,* Case No. CU-07-00204, San Benito County Superior Court (California), March 19, 2009.

7. Schmid.

8. California Department of Food and Agriculture. "New Coliform Bacteria Standard for California Raw Milk Producers." Press release (October 26, 2007). Available online at www.cdfa.ca.gov/egov/Press_Releases/Press_Release.asp?PRnum=07-090. Accessed May 2, 2009.

9. California Department of Food and Agriculture. "New Coliform Standard for Milk Sold Raw to Consumers" (January 2008). Available online at www.cdfa.ca.gov/AHFSS/Milk_and_Dairy_Food_Safety/pdfs/ColiformStandardMilkConsumedRaw.pdf. Accessed May 2, 2009.

10. www.thecompletepatient.com/journal/2007/11/7/the-other-ca-dairy-speaks-out-they-seem-to-want-to-totally-d.html. Accessed May 2, 2009.

11. www.thecompletepatient.com/journal/2007/11/1/not-so-fast-as-key-ca-ag-legislator-vows-to-protect-us-wante.html. Accessed May 2, 2009.

12. *Herzog v. Organic Pastures Dairy Company, LLC,* Case No. 08CECG00421, Fresno County Superior Court (California), February 6, 2008. Available online at www.marlerblog.com/Herzog%20-%20Complaint.PDF. Accessed May 2, 2009.

13. *Martin and McGonigle-Martin v. Organic Pastures Dairy Company, LLC,* Case No. 08CECG00408, Fresno County Superior Court (California), February 6, 2008. Available online at www.marlerblog.com/Martin%20-%20Complaint.PDF. Accessed May 2, 2009.

14. *Organic Pastures Dairy Company, LLC and Claravale Farm, Inc. v. State of California and A. G. Kawamura,* Case No. CU-07-00204, San Benito County Superior Court (California), December 27, 2007. Available online at www.ftcldf.org/litigation/ca-raw-milk/complaint_as_filed_1-0.pdf. Accessed May 2, 2009.

15. www.thecompletepatient.com/journal/2008/1/3/in-ca-ab-1735-conflict-you-cant-tell-the-players-or-the-play.html. Accessed May 2, 2009.

16. www.youtube.com/watch?v=jDh6Oqw7ZEs. Accessed May 2, 2009.

17. www.youtube.com/watch?v=_IdfYZcxZPk&NR=1. Accessed May 2, 2009.

18. Affidavit of Mark McAfee in *Organic Pastures Dairy Company, LLC and Claravale Farm, Inc. v. State of California and A. G. Kawamura,* Case No. CU-07-00204, San Benito County Superior Court (California), February 2008. Available online at www.ftcldf.org/litigation/ca-raw-milk/Aff_of_Mark_McAfee_on_lined_pap_11-0.pdf. Accessed May 2, 2009.

19. www.thecompletepatient.com/journal/2008/1/1/forget-the-ca-happy-talk-says-aajonus-vonderplanitz-he-promi.html. Accessed May 2, 2009.

20. www.thecompletepatient.com/journal/2007/11/19/the-story-behind-the-story-of-ron-pauls-raw-milk-proposal-ar.html. Accessed May 2, 2009.

21. Affidavit of Theodore Beals in *Organic Pastures Dairy Company, LLC and Claravale Farm, Inc. v. State of California and A. G. Kawamura,* Case No. CU-07-00204, San Benito County Superior Court (California), February 2008. Available online at www.ftcldf.org/litigation/ca-raw-milk/Affidavit_of_Ted_Beals_(correct_7-0.pdf. Accessed May 2, 2009.

22. Opposition to Application for Temporary Restraining Order in *Organic Pastures Dairy Company, LLC and Claravale Farm, Inc. v. State of California and A. G. Kawamura,* Case No. CU-07-00204, San Benito County Superior Court (California), March 12, 2008. Available online at www.thecompletepatient.com/storage/CAAGargument.pdf. Accessed May 2, 2009.

23. www.thecompletepatient.com/journal/2008/3/20/of-nighttime-agent-visits-phone-tapes-and-secret-wires-now-o.html. Accessed May 2, 2009.

24. www.thecompletepatient.com/journal/2008/4/16/sen-florezs-message-to-raw-milk-community-theres-no-going-ba.html. Accessed May 2, 2009.

25. California Senate Bill No. 201 (2008). *Dairy Farms: Raw Milk: Testing: Standards.* Available online at www.centralvalleybusinesstimes.com/links/sb_201_bill_20080902_enrolled.pdf. Accessed May 2, 2009.

26. http://haphazardgourmet.blogspot.com/2008/09/martin-sheen-is-gentleman-at-raw-milk.html. Accessed May 2, 2009.

27. www.marlerblog.com/2008/08/articles/case-news/governor-schwarzenegger-veto-this-bill. Accessed May 2, 2009.

28. Marler, Bill. "Organic Pastures *E. coli* O157:H7 2006 Outbreak" (2009). Available online at www.marlerblog.com/uploads/file/Organic%20Pastures%202006%20Outbreak.pdf. Accessed May 2, 2009.

Chapter 12: A Test of Belief Systems

1. www.thecompletepatient.com/journal/2008/9/11/how-much-punishment-is-enough-for-a-couples-tainted-raw-milk.html. Accessed May 3, 2009.
2. Complaint for Permanent Injunction in *United States of America v. Organic Pastures Dairy Company, LLC and Mark McAfee*, Case No. 1:08-at-00692, US District Court for the Eastern District of California, November 20, 2008. Available online at www .thecompletepatient.com/storage/US%20Complaint%20for%20Permanent%20 Injunction.pdf. Accessed May 3, 2009.
3. Farm-to-Consumer Legal Defense Fund announcement. "FDA Files Civil Lawsuit Against Organic Pastures Dairy." Available online at www.farmtoconsumer.org/ news/news-24nov2008.htm. Accessed July 2, 2009.
4. Sheehan, John F. "On the Safety of Raw Milk (With a Word About Pasteurization)." Slide 67 of slide-show presentation (May 12, 2005). Available online at www.cfsan .fda.gov/~ear/milksafe/milksa67.htm. Accessed May 3, 2009.
5. www.thecompletepatient.com/journal/2009/4/19/wherein-i-try-to-deal-with-this-obsession-does-fda-milk-czar.html. Accessed May 3, 2009.
6. Greer, William R. "Raw Milk Is Curbed." *New York Times* (January 7, 1987). Available online at www.nytimes.com/1987/01/07/garden/raw-milk-is-curbed. html?n=Top/Reference/Times%20Topics/Subjects/M/Milk. Accessed May 3, 2009.
7. Barrett, Stephen. "Why Raw Milk Should Be Avoided" (December 22, 2003). Available online at www.quackwatch.com/01QuackeryRelatedTopics/rawmilk.html. Accessed May 3, 2009.
8. Jarvis, William T. "Raw Milk Can Be Deadly" (1997). Available online at www.ncahf .org/articles/o-r/rawmilk.html. Accessed May 3, 2009.
9. www.law.georgetown.edu/faculty/facinfo/tab_faculty.cfm?Status=Faculty&ID=326. Accessed May 3, 2009.
10. US Constitution, Article I, section 10, clause 1. "Contract Clause." Available online at http://en.wikipedia.org/wiki/Contract_Clause. Accessed May 3, 2009.
11. www.thecompletepatient.com/journal/2008/8/13/ny-hearing-officer-to-smiths-raw-milk-is-raw-milk-whether-it.html. Accessed May 3, 2009.
12. www.thecompletepatient.com/journal/2008/11/24/state-judge-to-meadowsweet-its-ny-ag-markets-uber-alles-barb.html. Accessed May 3, 2009.
13. http://gov.ca.gov/pdf/press/SB201_Florez_Veto_Message.pdf. Accessed May 3, 2009.
14. www.miffs.org/MIfuwmilk/index.htm. Accessed May 3, 2009.
15. www.thecompletepatient.com/journal/2008/11/14/a-food-regulators-view-of-the-dangers-of-raw-milk-part-2-a-p.html. Accessed May 3, 2009.
16. Hadjigeorgalis, Ereney. "The US Dairy Industry and International Trade in Dairy Products" (September 2005). Available online at http://aces.nmsu.edu/pubs/ research/dairy/TR-42.pdf. Accessed May 3, 2009.
17. US Food and Drug Administration. "Grade 'A' Pasteurized Milk Ordinance, 2005 Revision." Available online at www.cfsan.fda.gov/~ear/pmo05toc.html. Accessed May 3, 2009.

18. www.thecompletepatient.com/journal/2009/2/9/connecticuts-raw-milk-proponents-mount-a-counter-offensive-t.html. Accessed May 3, 2009.
19. Prelli, F. Philip. "Legislature Must Rein in Risk of Raw Milk." Editorial. *Hartford Courant* (April 3, 2008).
20. www.thecompletepatient.com/journal/2009/4/6/sore-loser-did-the-fda-ghost-write-the-connecticut-ag-chiefs.html. Accessed May 3, 2009.
21. Drape, Joe. "Should This Milk Be Legal?" *New York Times* (August 8, 2007). Available online at www.nytimes.com/2007/08/08/dining/08raw.html?_r=1&scp=1&sq=raw%20milk&st=cse. Accessed July 2, 2009.
22. Monroe, Ann. "Trafficking in Raw Milk" (March 2009). Available online at http://lifestyle.msn.com/your-life/living-green/articlegreenchan.aspx?cp-documentid=18708415. Accessed May 3, 2009.

INDEX

ABOUT THE AUTHOR

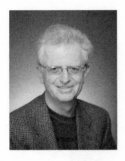 **David E. Gumpert** is a journalist who specializes in covering the intersection of health and business. His popular blog, www.thecompletepatient.com, has chronicled the increasingly unsettling battles over raw milk. He has authored or coauthored seven books on various aspects of entrepreneurship and business and previously been a reporter and editor with *Inc.* magazine, *The Wall Street Journal,* and *Harvard Business Review.*

Called "the high priest of the pasture" by *The New York Times,* foreword contributor **Joel Salatin** likes to refer to himself as a "Christian-libertarian-environmentalist-lunatic farmer." He lives with his family on Polyface Farm in the Shenandoah Valley of Virginia. He and his farm have been extensively profiled, including in Michael Pollan's *The Omnivore's Dilemma* and the documentary film *Food, Inc.* Salatin is the author of several books including *You Can Farm, Pastured Poultry Profits,* and *Everything I Want to Do Is Illegal.*

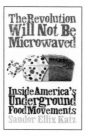
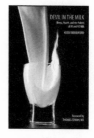
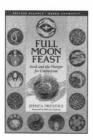
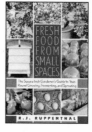
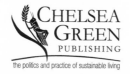